Current Topics in Environmental Health and Preventive Medicine

Series Editor

Takemi Otsuki
Kurashiki, Japan

Current Topics in Environmental Health and Preventive Medicine, published in partnership with the Japanese Society of Hygiene, is designed to deliver well written volumes authored by experts from around the globe, covering the prevention and environmental health related to medical, biological, molecular biological, genetic, physical, psychosocial, chemical, and other environmental factors. The series will be a valuable resource to both new and established researchers, as well as students who are seeking comprehensive information on environmental health and health promotion.

More information about this series at http://www.springer.com/series/13556

Masakazu Washio • Gen Kobashi
Editors

Epidemiological Studies of Specified Rare and Intractable Disease

Springer

Editors
Masakazu Washio
St. Mary's College
Kurume
Fukuoka
Japan

Gen Kobashi
Dokkyo Medical University
Mibu
Tochigi
Japan

ISSN 2364-8333 ISSN 2364-8341 (electronic)
Current Topics in Environmental Health and Preventive Medicine
ISBN 978-981-13-1095-9 ISBN 978-981-13-1096-6 (eBook)
https://doi.org/10.1007/978-981-13-1096-6

Library of Congress Control Number: 2018951099

This Springer imprint is published by the registered company Springer Nature Singapore Pte Ltd.
The registered company address is: 152 Beach Road, #21-01/04 Gateway East, Singapore 189721, Singapore

Preface

"Nanbyo" (i.e., rare intractable diseases) may be a heavy burden not only on the patients but also on their family members because these diseases have few established therapies yet, usually develop chronically, and often lead to great disabilities. The Japanese government has been promoting research on the etiology and treatment of "Nanbyo" in order to detect the causes of these diseases. Consequently, several epidemiological studies have revealed new findings, which suggest clues to understand the pathogeneses of "Nanbyo."

We are glad to have the great opportunity to introduce these findings through this book. We hope that this book will serve as one of the useful resources for all healthcare workers who treat and care "Nanbyo," as well as researchers who are interested in "Nanbyo" and its epidemiology.

Kurume, Fukuoka, Japan — Masakazu Washio
Mibu, Tochigi, Japan — Gen Kobashi

Contents

Chapter 1
Introduction of Epidemiological Studies of "Nanbyo"

Masakazu Washio and Yutaka Inaba

Abstract "Nanbyo" in Japanese is commonly used in the Japanese society to refer to so-called "intractable diseases." In this chapter, we would like to introduce "Nanbyo" and the role of the Research Committee of the Epidemiology of "Nanbyo." In 1972, the Japanese government began systemic countermeasures against "Nanbyo." Since then, the government has been promoting research on "Nanbyo." The Research Committee of the Epidemiology of "Nanbyo" was first organized in 1976. Because "Nanbyo" are diseases of low incidence and patients are scattered all over Japan, epidemiologists and clinicians work together to prevent laborious work as well as to save cost, and epidemiologists have many precious experiences by working with clinicians. Furthermore, younger epidemiologists are able to learn how to conduct epidemiological studies from senior epidemiologists of other universities and research institutes all over Japan. Although the involvement of epidemiologists was much lower in Japan than in the United Kingdom and the United States, based on the success experience of "Nanbyo," the government promotes collaborative studies with epidemiologists and clinicians to investigate not only "Nanbyo" but also other research subjects.

Keywords Nanbyo (intractable diseases) · Epidemiology

M. Washio (✉)
Department of Community Health and Clinical Epidemiology, St. Mary's College, Kurume City, Fukuoka, Japan
e-mail: washiomasa@yahoo.co.jp

Y. Inaba
Department of Epidemiology and Environmental Health, Juntendo University Faculty of Medicine, Bunkyo-ku, Tokyo, Japan
e-mail: yinaba@juntendo.ac.jp

M. Washio, G. Kobashi (eds.), *Epidemiological Studies of Specified Rare and Intractable Disease*, Current Topics in Environmental Health and Preventive Medicine, https://doi.org/10.1007/978-981-13-1096-6_1

1.1 What Is "Nanbyo"?

"Nanbyo" in Japanese is commonly used in the Japanese society to refer to so-called "intractable diseases," diseases which are not medically or clearly defined [1, 2]. Since the diagnosis of "intractable diseases" may depend on the level of health care and the social state of affairs in a country at that time, infectious diseases such as dysentery, cholera, and tuberculosis were categorized as "intractable diseases" at a time when there was neither sufficient health care nor effective treatment in Japan.

Improvement of public health and advances in medicine after World War II have given Japan one of the highest life expectancies in the world (i.e., 80.8 years old for men and 87.1 years old for women in 2015) [2]. With dramatically improved health care and medical care, the abovementioned infectious diseases can now be treated, and are no longer considered intractable. However, some diseases remain difficult to treat and easily become chronic; these are the kind of diseases that are now referred to as "Nanbyo" in Japan [1, 2]. According to the definition of "Nanbyo" published by the Japanese Ministry of Health and Welfare in 1972 [1, 2], "Nanbyo" refers to:

(1) diseases whose cause has not yet been detected and for which there is no established therapy, and which may have a considerably high risk of disability (e.g., Behçet's disease, myasthenia gravis, aplastic anemia, and malignant rheumatoid arthritis) [1, 2],
and
(2) diseases that chronically developed and require a significant amount of labor for the patient's care, causing a heavy burden on other family members of the patient, both financially and mentally (e.g., pediatric cancer, pediatric chronic nephritis, pediatric asthma, progressive muscular dystrophy, and renal insufficiency of dialysis patients) [1, 2].

1.2 Measures against "Nanbyo"

After World War II, in Japan, acute infectious diseases decreased with the improvement of public health and the progress in medicine while chronic diseases such as cancers and cardiovascular diseases increased [2]. Although various countermeasures were taken against cancers, cardiovascular diseases, infantile chronic diseases, and severe mental and physical disabilities, a national counterplan against "Nanbyo" was not sufficiently systematized due to obscure etiologies and strange clinical features [3].

Subacute myelo-optico-neuropathy (SMON), which was prevalent throughout Japan towards the end of 1960s, was the first "Nanbyo" in Japan [2–5]. The Japanese government organized task-force research groups for SMON consisting of clinicians, pathologists, neurologists, microbiologists, chemists, pharmacologists, epidemiologists, and other specialists [4], and the research groups reported that administration of clioquinol, a gastrointestinal disinfectant, might have played an important role in Japan in the development of SMON after World War II [4–9]. Meade [9] reported a hypothesis that combination of clioquinol and some environmental factor increased with postwar environmental pollution, which was much more widely distributed and in higher concentration in Japan than other countries, work together to increase the risk of SMON in Japan after World War II. His hypothesis may partly explain the reason why the incidence of SMON was much higher in Japan than in other countries [9], as well as the reason why there was no dose-response relationship between the administration of clioquinol and the severity of SMON [9].

In 1972, the Japanese government started systemic countermeasures against "Nanbyo" [2–4], which were eight intractable diseases including SMON (Table 1.1). Since 1972, the Japanese government has been promoting research on the etiology and treatment of "Nanbyo." The Research Committee of the Epidemiology of "Nanbyo" was first organized in 1976 [2, 3].

Besides promotion of survey/research on "Nanbyo," other measures against "Nanbyo" are (1) establishment of medical institutions for "Nanbyo," (2) reduction of co-payment of medical fees for "Nanbyo," (3) improvement and cooperation in community-based health care, medical care, and welfare services for patients with "Nanbyo," and (4) promotion of welfare measures in order to improve quality of life of patients with "Nanbyo" [2].

The number of Japanese government-certified "Nanbyo" increased from eight diseases in 1972 to 330 diseases in 2017 [10]. In the New Measures against "Nanbyo" started from 2015, the Japanese government reviewed and decided designated intractable diseases to support medical expenses as Japanese government-certified "Nanbyo" [10].

As shown in Table 1.2, the criteria for "Nanbyo" are as follows: (1) unknown etiology, (2) lack of effective treatment, (3) rare disease, and (4) necessity of long-term care [9]. In addition to the above four criterions, the designated intractable diseases are required to meet two additional criterions: (5) the prevalence of the disease must be less than 0.1% of the Japanese population and (6) the disease must have objective diagnostic criteria [10].

Table 1.1 Japanese government-certified "Nanbyo" in 1972

1. Subacute myelo-optico-neuropathy(SMON)
2. Behçet's disease
3. Myasthenia gravis
4. Systemic lupus erythematosus
5. Sarcoidosis
6. Aplastic anemia
7. Multiple sclerosis
8. Fulminant hepatitis

Table 1.2 The criteria for "Nanbyo" (intractable diseases)

1. Unknown etiology
2. Lack of effective treatment
3. Rare disease
4. Necessity of long-term care
Additional two criterions for the designated intractable diseases
5. Prevalence of the disease is less than 0.1% of the Japanese population
6. The disease has objective diagnostic criteria

1.3 Epidemiology of "Nanbyo"

1.3.1 Epidemiological Studies of "Nanbyo"

Epidemiology is the study of the distribution and determinants of health-related states or events (i.e., death, disease, discomfort, disability, dissatisfaction) in specified populations, and the application of this study to the control of diseases and other health problems [11, 12]. The established diagnosis criterion is needed to carry out the epidemiological studies of "Nanbyo."

Epidemiological studies are classified as either observational studies or experimental studies [11, 12]. Since observational studies allow nature to take its course [11, 12], epidemiologists observe without intervention other than record, classify, count, and statistically analyze results [11, 12]. Japanese epidemiologists conducted observational studies of "Nanbyo" because "Nanbyo" are diseases whose cause is unknown and for which there is no established therapy [1, 2, 13].

Observational epidemiological studies comprise both descriptive epidemiological studies and analytical epidemiological studies [11]. Descriptive epidemiological studies are conducted to investigate the course of "Nanbyo" as well as to estimate the frequency and distribution of the patients with "Nanbyo" by the statistics of patients receiving financial aid for treatment, national patient surveys and nationwide hospital surveys [13].

Since the prevalence of "Nanbyo" was low and the patients were scattered throughout Japan, epidemiologists, who were engaged in the research on the first eight "Nanbyo" (i.e., SMON, Behçet's disease, myasthenia gravis, systemic lupus erythematosus, sarcoidosis, aplastic anemia, multiple sclerosis, and fulminant hepatitis), planned to coordinate their work by nationwide surveys of these eight diseases in order to obtain basic data of the patients [4, 13]. With the increase in the number of Japanese government-certified "Nanbyo," nationally surveyed "Nanbyo" increased afterwards as well.

The nationwide epidemiological survey of "Nanbyo" consists of the primary survey for the estimation of number of patients with the target intractable disease and the second survey for the recognition of their clinical and epidemiological features [14].

In the primary survey, all hospitals with 200 beds or more were asked to answer how many male and female patients with the target intractable disease they treated by mail until 1992 [14]. Since 1993, sample surveys have been chosen for the nationwide epidemiological survey of "Nanbyo" in Japan [14]. In the sample surveys, the facilities of the target intractable disease are randomly chosen from hospitals all over Japan according to the scale of the hospitals at a certain extraction rate (i.e., 100% for medical school hospitals, 100% for general hospitals with 500 beds or more, 80% for general hospitals with 400–499 beds, 40% for general hospitals with 300–399 beds, 20% for general hospitals with 200–299 beds, 10% for general hospitals with 100–199 beds, 5% for general hospitals with 99 beds or less, and 100% for special hospitals regardless of hospital scale) [15]. In most cases, special hospitals are hospitals where patients with the target intractable disease are concentrated on because the members of clinical research committee of the target intractable diseases and/or the councilors of the academic society of the target intractable diseases treat these patients as clinicians [15]. Therefore, the nationwide epidemiological survey of "Nanbyo" may avoid missing the important information about patients with the target intractable disease in the small scale of hospitals after the introduction of the sample survey methods.

In the second survey, the research group sent self-administrated questionnaires to each hospital that stated that they treated one or more patients with the target intractable disease in order to obtain information about each of their patients (i.e., sex, age, present address, job, medical insurance, public financial aid for treatment and disease activities such as disability certificate, and clinical characteristics) to be surveyed nationwide [14].

From fiscal years 1988 to 1992, research groups of epidemiologists estimated the number of patients with over 40 target intractable diseases [13].

After fiscal year 1993, numerous nationwide epidemiological surveys were conducted to estimate the number of patients with "Nanbyo" by the sample survey methods. Among them, we would like to introduce several findings of our research team. In 1999, Nakagawa et al. [16] estimated the annual numbers of patients by type of AL amyloidosis, AA amyloidosis, and amyloidosis in patients on hemodialysis were 510 (95% confidence interval: 410–620), 1800 (95% confidence interval: 700–2900), and 4500 (95% confidence interval: 3400–5600), which revealed that the number of amyloidosis in hemodialysis patients increased compared with that of former survey, owing to the elongation of the period of hemodialysis. On the other hand, Lin et al. [17] estimated that the annual number of patients with acute pancreatitis was 19,500 (95% confidence interval: 17,000–22,000) from the first survey and reported that the sex ratio (male/female) was 1.9 among 1688 patients and 87 patients (21.4%) died among 409 severe acute pancreatic patients from the second survey in 1999. In 2005, Kurosawa et al. [18] estimated that the annual number of patients with Behçet's disease was 15,000 (95% confidence interval: 14,000–16,000) from the first survey conducted in 2002, and found that the number of patients in 2002 was smaller than the number of patients in 1991 (i.e., 18,400), but greater than the number of patients in 1984, 1979, and 1972 (i.e., 13,000, 11,500, and 8500). The second survey, which was conducted in 2003, revealed that only 0.7% of patients with Behçet's disease were almost always hospitalized while 86.5% of patients with Behçet's disease were outpatients in Japan [18]. The proportion of the patients who were almost always hospitalized decreased from 10% in 1972 to 0.7% in 2003 [18].

The nationwide epidemiological surveys of "Nanbyo" give us not only the estimated number of patients with the target intractable diseases, but also changes in the numbers and prognosis of these patients, as well as the quality of life of these patients [14]. Findings from the nationwide epidemiological surveys of "Nanbyo" have given us important information as to how we should support patients with "Nanbyo" in Japan.

Nationwide epidemiological surveys were conducted for estimating the number of patients with intractable diseases whose disease were not certified by the Japanese government. Tamakoshi et al. [19] conducted nationwide epidemiological surveys of intractable diseases with no subsidy for treatment in 1999. They estimated the number of patients with over 40 intractable diseases without any subsidy for treatment such as primary hyperlipidemia (83,270, 95% confidence interval: 43,930–122,610), Guillain–Barré syndrome (2500, 95% confidence interval: 2000–2900), and Fabry disease (150, 95% confidence interval: 95–205) [19].

However, they could not conduct nationwide epidemiological surveys of several "Nanbyo" without the established diagnosis criterion [19].

Epidemiologists should remember that the established diagnosis criterion of the target disease is necessary to carry out nationwide epidemiological surveys. Nowadays, polyneuropathy with monoclonal gammopathy provides the established diagnosis criterion as the polyneuropathy, organomegaly, endocrinopathy, monoclonal gammopathy, and skin changes (POEMS) syndrome and is treated as one of the government-certified intractable diseases in Japan [1].

Besides nationwide surveys, epidemiological studies using the records of patients who have registered for public financial aid have provided useful information regarding "Nanbyo" in Japan. Ohta et al. [20] investigated peak onset ages of "Nanbyo" using the clinical database of 216,160 patients with "Nanbyo" receiving public financial aid for treatment in 2003. They found that the distribution of ages at onset and peak onset ages could be systematically clarified for each kind of "Nanbyo" [20]. Peak onset ages were under 20 years for primary immune deficiency syndrome, subacute sclerosing panencephalitis, lysosomal diseases, epidermolysis bullosa, and neurofibromatosis I and II, while aortitis syndrome, SLE, Behçet's disease, adrenoleukodystrophy, multiple sclerosis, ulcerative colitis, and Crohn's disease showed peak onset ages between 20 and 50 years [20]. On the other hand, distributions of onset ages were bimodal for aplastic anemia, idiopathic thrombocytopenic purpura, myasthenia gravis, moyamoya disease, and sarcoidosis [20], and many other intractable diseases showed peak onset ages of older than 40 years [20]. Their study provides information about the natural history of development of each intractable disease in Japan [20].

Using case cards of "Nanbyo" patients recorded on magnetic tape obtained from the Ministry of Health and Welfare, Inaba et al. [21] estimated the number of patients with the target intractable diseases in the National One-day Patient Survey of "Nanbyo." In the National One-day Patient Survey of "Nanbyo," each patient survey was conducted through medical institutions selected by stratified sampling in terms of type of institution, such as hospitals or general clinics, and prefecture [21]. These selected medical institutions were asked to report the number of patients who received medical treatment on a specified day [21].

Table 1.3 shows three kinds of estimate number of patients with the first eight Japanese government-certified "Nanbyo" around 1990 [21]. The nationwide surveys were excellent in diagnosis of each of the "Nanbyo," but they were usually carried out using only the hospitals with more than 200 beds at these years before 1993 [14, 21], and the response rates were around 50% [21]. The National One-day Patient Survey is carried out with more statistically restricted plan using all hospitals and clinics [21]. However, there is a serious limitation in the National One-day Patient Survey because the individual patient forms for the survey are fulfilled in by persons other than physicians in many institutions. Moreover, the studied diseases are classified by ICD code and some "Nanbyo" are impossible to fit into the exact code. The data of patients receiving financial aid for treatment is not estimated but real data. However, there are two limitations: (1) elderly patients who have other financial aid may not apply for this aid and (2) evaluation of the applicant is based on different standards among the 47 prefectures [21].

On the other hand, there are four major analytical epidemiological studies, which are cohort studies, case-control studies, cross-sectional studies, and ecological studies [11]. Among the four major analytical epidemiological studies, cohort studies, in which subjects free of the disease in a source population are classified into subgroups according to exposure to a potential cause of the disease, provide the best information about the causation of the disease but may require observation of large numbers over long periods [11]. On the other hand, case-control studies are relatively simple and economical to carry out and are used to investigate causes of diseases, especially rare disease [11]. In case-control studies,

Table 1.3 Estimate number of patients with the first eight Japanese government-certified "Nanbyo" around 1990 [21]

The name of diseases	Estimated number of patients		Registered number of patients in financial aid for treatment in 1990
	By Nationwide survey (study year)	By National One-day Patient Survey in 1993	
1. Subacute myelo-optico-neuropathy (SMON)	14,600 (1980)	Not available	2201
2. Behçet's disease	12,000–15,000 (1984)	12,407–17,320	11,890
3. Myasthenia gravis	5000–7000 (1986)	6530–10,957	6929
4. Systemic lupus erythematosus	20,000–25,600 (1989)	29,417–35,782	29,594
5. Sarcoidosis	3000–7500 (1984)	7981–12,435	6939
6. Aplastic anemia	4000–6200 (1982)	6884–10,095	6618
7. Multiple sclerosis	2000–4500 (1984)	4604–7987	3212
8. Fulminant hepatitis	Not available	8820–15,666	Not available

cases are subjects with the disease of interest while control subjects are a suitable comparison group of people unaffected by the disease [11]. Since Japanese government-certified "Nanbyo" are rare intractable diseases [10], Japanese epidemiologists have carried out numerous case-control studies to promote the elucidation of the causes of "Nanbyo" in the Research Committee of the Epidemiology of "Nanbyo" [13].

Cross-sectional studies measure the prevalence of disease and the prevalence of risk/preventive factors at the same time [11]. Using similar methods to those for case-control studies, epidemiologists can investigate the association between the disease and exposures in cross-sectional studies, which are relatively easy and economical to carry out [11]. The nationwide cross-sectional study revealed that both anti-centromere antibody and anti-topoisomerase I antibody showed a positive association with lung fibrosis in patients with systemic sclerosis receiving financial aid for treatment in Japan [22].

Cross-sectional studies of "Nanbyo" are also carried out to investigate the need of social services among patients with "Nanbyo" [23, 24].

Ecological studies usually rely on data collected for other purposes, where the units of analysis are groups of people rather than individuals [11]. Although ecological studies are easy to carry out, the association observed between variables at the group levels doses not necessarily represent the association that exists at the individual levels [11]. However, ecological studies are useful epidemiologic tools for public health if we know the limitations of ecological studies and interpret the results carefully. Morbidities and the utilizations of social services/medical payment in different prefectures as well as in the nationwide surveys at different time may give us useful information for measures against "Nanbyo."

1.3.2 The Research Committee of the Epidemiology of "Nanbyo"

Since 1976, the Research Committee of the Epidemiology of "Nanbyo" conducted epidemiological studies with the cooperation of public health centers, medical school hospitals, and other flagship hospitals [13]. Because "Nanbyo" are diseases with a low incidence and patients with "Nanbyo" are scattered all over Japan, epidemiologists and clinicians in the study teams conduct case-control studies together to save laborious work and cost as well as to detect factors related to the development of "Nanbyo" [4]. In addition, nationwide surveys of "Nanbyo" have been carried out by the Research Committee of the Epidemiology of "Nanbyo" in cooperation with clinical research groups (i.e., doctors working at medical school hospitals or flagship hospitals) [13]. Therefore, epidemiologists have been able to have many valuable experiences by working with clinicians in the Research Committee of the Epidemiology of "Nanbyo" [4]. Furthermore, younger epidemiologists learn how to conduct epidemiological studies of "Nanbyo" from senior epidemiologists of other universities and research institutes all over Japan.

1.3.3 How a Young Epidemiologist Learned the Epidemiology of "Nanbyo" in the Research Committee of the Epidemiology

Masakazu Washio: In 1999, I joined in the Research Committee of the Epidemiology of "Nanbyo" (Chairman. Prof. Yutaka Inaba, Juntendo University). At that time, I was a physician of a geriatric hospital as well as a part-time research fellow epidemiologist of Kyushu University. Prof. Heizo Tanaka, who was a professor of the Medical Research Institute Tokyo Medical and Dental University as well as the Editor-in-Chief of official journal of Japan Epidemiological Association, allowed young epidemiologists to join in his research project (i.e., case-control studies of risk and preventive factors for so-called intractable diseases) [25] . In this research team, we reviewed research papers on risk factors for inflammatory bowel diseases, ossification of the posterior longitudinal ligament of the spines (OPLL), and systemic lupus erythematosus (SLE). As coworkers, we planned to evaluate both environmental and genetic factors.

In 2000, Dr. Gen Kobashi planned to carry out a case-control study to detect environmental and genetic risk factors for OPLL [26]. I asked orthopedists of university hospitals in Kyushu to join as coworkers in our study. Later, I had the opportunity to write a research paper on the lifestyle factors and the risk of OPLL in Japan [27].

In 2002, I became a partaker of the Research Committee of the Epidemiology of "Nanbyo" (Chairman. Prof. Yutaka Inaba, Juntendo University) and planned to carry out a case control study to evaluate environmental and genetic risk factors for SLE [28], which was referred to as the Kyushu Sapporo SLE (KYSS) study. At this time, I worked as educational staff at the Department of the Public Health, Sapporo Medical University.

The experience of the previous case-control study of OPLL in the Research Committee of the Epidemiology of "Nanbyo" (Chairman. Prof. Yutaka Inaba, Juntendo University) [28] was very helpful for me to make a study design to evaluate environmental and genetic risk factors for SLE.

From 2005 to 2011, I continued to carry out case control studies of "Nanbyo" as a member of the Research Committee of the Epidemiology of "Nanbyo" (Chairman. Prof. Masaki Nagai, Saitama Medical University) although I moved to St. Mary's College in 2006. Even after the Research Committee of the Epidemiology of "Nanbyo" (Chairman. Prof. Masaki Nagai, Saitama Medical University) ended, I continued with the Kyushu Sapporo SLE (KYSS) study as a project leader.

Through working as a member of the Research Committee of the Epidemiology of "Nanbyo," I learned how to work together with the epidemiologists and clinicians of other institutes in our research project (i.e., the KYSS study). According to the advice of seniors, I put together a small research team so that I could identify the face, name, and specialty of each coworker in the KYSS study. The KYSS study was a case-control study to evaluate environmental and genetic risk factors for SLE among Japanese females. SLE patients were recruited from female outpatients of Kyushu University Hospital, Saga University Hospital, and their collaborating hospitals in Kyushu, while SLE patients were female outpatients recruited from Sapporo Medical University Hospital and Hokkaido University Hospital in Hokkaido [29, 30]. All patients fulfilled the American College of Rheumatology 1982 revised criteria for SLE [31]. Controls were recruited from nursing college students and care workers in nursing homes in Kyushu while in Hokkaido controls were recruited from female participants of a health checkup in a local town. A self-administered questionnaire was obtained from SLE patients and controls, along with written informed consent for cooperation in the study. A section of the participants also agreed to donate blood samples, which were stored until use for DNA extraction and genotyping of the candidate genes of SLE [29, 30].

Both epidemiologists and clinicians published research papers on risk factors for SLE in this study project. Smoking [29, 30, 32–34], stress [32], history of surgery [30], history of blood transfusion [30], family history of SLE [34], family history of connective tissue disease [34], and intake of dairy products [35], coffee [36], and black tea [36] were associated with an increased risk of SLE while light/moderate alcohol consumption [33] and live childbirth [30] were suggested to decrease the risk of SLE. On the other hand, association of the polymorphisms of the genes, the individuals carrying two or more "at-risk" genotypes of TNF receptor type II gene (TNF-RII), cytochrome P4501A1 gene (CYP1A1) and glutathione S-transferase M1 gene (GSTM1) had a significantly increased risk for SLE compared with those having each "at-risk" genotype [37]. Further studies are needed to confirm the findings of the KYSS study.

1.4 Conclusion

Nowadays, research projects on overcoming "Nanbyo" (Grant-in-aid research) are conducted to investigate the causes of "Nanbyo" as well as to develop groundbreaking methods of diagnosis and treatment of "Nanbyo."

Although the involvement of epidemiologists is much lower in Japan compared with the United Kingdom and the United States [38], the Research Committee of the Epidemiology of "Nanbyo" has given epidemiologists the opportunity to investigate "Nanbyo" with clinicians, which may help Japanese clinicians to understand an important role of epidemiology in clinical studies. Based on the success experience of the Research Committee of the Epidemiology of "Nanbyo," the Japanese government promotes collaborative studies with epidemiologists and clinicians to investigate not only "Nanbyo" but also other research subjects, such as the prevention of pneumonia in the elderly [39, 40].

References

1. Japan Intractable Disease Information Center. What is an intractable disease? http://www.nanbyou.or.jp/english/index.htm. Accessed 2 July, 2015.
2. Health, Labour and Welfare Statistics Association. Trend of national health 2016–2017. Tokyo: Health, Labour and Welfare Statistics Association. 2016. (in Japanese).
3. Yoshitoshi Y. Countermeasures agaist intractable diseases in Japan. Jap J Med 17(1): 1–2, 1978. ONLINE ISSN: 1881-123X PRINT ISSN: 0021-5120
4. Aoki K, Shigematsu I. Epidemiological methods: a view from north Asia/Japan. In: Holland WW, Olsen J, du V. Florey C (eds) The development of modern epidemiology: personal reports from those who were there. Oxford University Press, Oxford, pp. 349–360; 2007.
5. Iwashita H. The history and present of SMON research in Japan. Iryo. 2001;55(10):510–5. (in Japanese)
6. Aoyama H, Ohira M, Yoshioka S, Ohta T, et al. Epidemiological sudies on subacute myelo-optico neuropathy (SMON) in the town of Yubara, Japan (report 4). Nihon Eiseigaku Zasshi. 1972;27(4):357–63. (in Japanese)
7. Kasai M. Subacute myelo-optico neuropathy (SMON) in Hokkaido, an epidemiological study (report 1). Nihon Eiseigaku Zasshi. 1973;28(3):315–23. (in Japanese)
8. Kuratusune M, Yoshimura T, Tokudome S, Kouchi S, Matsuzaka J. An epidemiological study on the association between SMON and chinoform. Nihon Eiseigaku Zasshi. 1973;28(5):450–5. (in Japanese)
9. Meade TW. Subacute myelo-optic neuropathy and clioquinol. An epidemiological case-history for diagnosis. Br J Prev Soc Med. 1975;29(3):157–69. PMID:127638
10. Japan Intractable Disease Information Center. New Measures against "Nanbyo" started from 2015. http://www.nanbyou.or.jp/entry/index.1441. Accessed 15 July, 2017. (in Japanese).
11. Beaglehole R, Bonita R, Kjellstroem T. Basic epidemiology. Geneva: World Health Organization; 1993.
12. Porta M, Greenland S, Last JM. A dictionary of epidemiology. 5th ed. Oxford: Oxford University Press; 2008.
13. Yanagawa H. Recent progress of epidemiological studies on intractable diseases in Japan. Nihon Eiseigaku Zasshi. 1995;49:950–9. (in Japanese)
14. Kawamura T. Significance of nation-wide epidemiological survey. In: Kawamura T (ed) Manual of nation-wide epidemiological survey for estimating the annual number of patients treated for intractable diseases and for recognizing their clinical features, 2nd edn. Research Committee on Epidemiology of Intractable Diseases, Ministry of Health and Welfare of Japan. pp 4–6; 2006. (in Japanese).
15. Tamakoshi A, Kawamura T. Procedure of nation-wide epidemiological survey. In: Kawamura T (ed) Manual of nationwide epidemiological survey for estimating the annual number of patients treated for intractable diseases and for recognizing their clinical features, 2nd edn. Research Committee on Epidemiology of Intractable Diseases, Ministry of Health and Welfare of Japan. pp 8–14; 2006. (in Japanese).
16. Nakagawa H, Morikawa Y, Mirura K, et al. Nation-wide epidemiological surve of amyloidosis. In: Inaba Y (ed) Annual report of research committee on epidemiology of intractable diseases, Ministry of Health and Welfare of Japan. pp 55–60; 2000. (in Japanese).
17. Lin Y, Tamakoshi A, Ohno Y, et al. Nation-wide epidemiological surve of acute pancreatitis in Japan. In: Inaba Y (eds) Annual report of research committee on epidemiology of intractable diseases, Ministry of Health and Welfare of Japan. pp 72–78; 2000. (in Japanese).
18. Kurosawa M, Inaba Y. A recent trend of epidemiological feature of Behçet's disease. Igakuno Ayumi. 2005; 215: 5–8. (in Japanese).

19. Tamakoshi A, Ohno Y, Kawamura T, Hashimoto S, Nagai M. Nationwide epidemiological survey of intractable diseases with no subsidy for treatment. Iryo. 2002;56(1):51–8.
20. Ohta A, Nagai M, Nishina M, et al. Age at the onset of intractable disease: based on a clinical database for patients receiving financial aid for treatment. Nihon Koshu Eisei Zasshi. 2007;54(1):3–14. (in Japanese)
21. Inaba Y, Minowa M, Osaki Y, et al. Recent statistical data book on intractable diseases in Japan. Research Committee on Epidemiology of Intractable Diseases, the Ministry of Health and Welfare of Japan; 1996.
22. Sakauchi F, Mori M, Ishikawa O, Endo H, Shinkai H. Epidemiological study on patients with systemic sclerosis receiving financial aid for treatment. Nihon Rinsho Meneki Gakkai Kaishi. 2003;26(2):66–73. (in Japanese)
23. Matsuba T, Inaba Y, Kurosawa M, et al. The study on the usages of health care and welfare services among patients with Parkinson's disease and their satisfaction levels. In: Inaba Y (ed) Annual report of research committee on epidemiology of intractable diseases, Ministry of Health, Labour and Welfare of Japan. pp 118–120; 2002. (in Japanese).
24. Matsushima A, Matsumoto A, Moriwaka F, et al. A cross-sectional study on socioeconomic systems supporting outpatients with Parkinson's disease in Japan. J Epidemiol. 2016;26(4):185–90. https://doi.org/10.2188/jea.JE20150081.
25. Tanaka H, Okamoto K, Kobashi G, et al. Case-control studies of risk and preventive factors for so-called intractable disease. In: Inaba Y (ed) Annual report of research committee on epidemiology of intractable diseases, Ministry of Health and Welfare of Japan. pp 9–15; 2000. (in Japanese).
26. Kobashi G, Okamoto K, Washio M, et al. A case-control study to detect lifestyle and genetic risk factors for ossification of the posterior longitudinal ligament of spines. In: Inaba Y (ed) Annual report of research committee on epidemiology of intractable diseases, Ministry of Health, Labour and Welfare of Japan. pp 17–19; 2001. (in Japanese).
27. Washio M, Kobashi G, Okamoto K, et al. Sleeping habit and other life styles in the prime of life and risk for ossification of the posterior longitudinal ligament of the spine (OPLL): a case-control study in Japan. J Epidemiol. 2004;14(5):168–73.
28. Washio M, Kiyohara C, Horiuchi T, et al. A case control study of systemic lupus erythematosus. In: Inaba Y (ed) Annual report of research committee on epidemiology of intractable diseases, Ministry of Health, Labour and Welfare of Japan. pp 10–12; 2003. (in Japanese).
29. Washio M, Horiuchi T, Kiyohara C, et al. Smoking, drinking, sleeping habits, and other lifestyle factors and the risk of systemic lupus erythematosus in Japanese females: findings from the KYSS study. Mod Rheumatol. 2006;16(3):143–50. https://doi.org/10.1007/s10165-006-0474-6.
30. Washio M, Takahashi H, Kobashi G, et al. Risk factors for development of systemic lupus erythematosus among Japanese females: medical history and reproductive factors. Int J Rheum Dis. 2017;20(1):76–83. https://doi.org/10.1111/1756-185X.12600.
31. Tan EM, Cohen AS, Fries JF, et al. The 1982 revised criteria for the classification of systemic lupus erythematosus. Arthritis Rheum. 1982;25(11):1271–7.
32. Takahashi H, Washio M, Kiyohara C, et al. Psychological stress in a Japanese population with systemic lupus erythematosus: finding from KYSS study. Mod Rheumatol. 2014;24(3):448–52. https://doi.org/10.3109/14397595.2013.843745.
33. Kiyohara C, Washio M, Horiuchi T, et al. Cigarette smoking, alcohol consumption, and risk of systemic lupus erythematosus: a case-control study in a Japanese population. J Rheumatol. 2012;39(7):1363–70. https://doi.org/10.3899/jrheum.111609.
34. Tada Y, Washio M, Horiuchi T, et al. Influence of medical history in parents or siblings on the development of systemic lupus Erythematosus among Japanese females. Int Med J. 2016;23(5):466–9. ISSN: 1341-2051
35. Kiyohara C, Washio M, Horiuchi T, et al. (2015) Dietary patterns and the risk of systemic lupus Erythematosus in a Japanese population: the Kyushu Sapporo SLE (KYSS) study. Int Med J, 22(3): 110–115. ISSN: 1341–2051.

36. Kiyohara C, Washio M, Horiuchi T, et al. Modifying effect of N-acetyltransferase 2 genotype on the association between systemic lupus erythematosus and consumption of alcohol and caffeine-rich beverages. Arthritis Care Res (Hoboken). 2014;66(7):1048–56. https://doi.org/10.1002/acr.22282.
37. Horiuchi T, Washio M, Kiyohara C, et al. Combination of TNF-RII, CYP1A1 and GSTM1 polymorphisms and the risk of Japanese SLE: findings from the KYSS study. Rheumatology (Oxford). 2009;48(9):1045–9. https://doi.org/10.1093/rheumatology/kep166.
38. Takahashi K, Washio M, Ren A, Tokui N, Aw TC, Wong O. An international comparison of the involvement of epidemiology in the most frequently cited publications in the field of clinical medicine. J Epidemiol. 2001;11(1):41–5.
39. Kondo K, Suzuki K, Washio M, et al. Association between monovalent influenza a (H1N1) pdm09 vaccine and pneumonia among the elderly in the 2009-2010 seasons in Japan: a case-control study. Hum Vaccin Immunother. 2015;11(5):1088–93. https://doi.org/10.1080/21645515.2015.1016668.
40. Washio M, Kondo K, Fujisawa N, et al. Hypoalbuminemia, influenza vaccination and other factors related to the development of pneumonia acquired outside hospitals in southern Japan: a case-control study. Geriatr Gerontol Int. 2016;16(2):223–9. https://doi.org/10.1111/ggi.12456.

Chapter 2
Risk Factors for Ossification of Posterior Longitudinal Ligament

Mitsumasa Umesawa, Koji Uchiyama, Hiroshi Taneichi, and Gen Kobashi

Abstract Ossification of the posterior longitudinal ligament (OPLL) is a kind of ectopic ossification occurred at the spinal canal. OPLL causes myeloradiculopathy. The prevalence of OPLL in Asian population is generally higher than in Western population. Also, the prevalence of OPLL is higher in older subjects than in younger subjects. Risk factors of OPLL were discussed by epidemiological studies. These studies found that genetic factors, obesity, history of diseases, and nutritional factors were likely to be risk factor of OPLL.

Keywords Ossification of the posterior longitudinal ligament (OPLL) · Epidemiology · Risk factor

2.1 Introduction

The ossification of the posterior longitudinal ligament (OPLL) is a type of ectopic ossification that occurs in the spinal canal. Patients are commonly asymptomatic during the early course of the disease. However, OPLL progression causes myeloradiculopathy because the ossified ligament continuously presses on the spinal cord and nerve roots.

M. Umesawa · G. Kobashi (✉)
Department of Public Health, Dokkyo Medical University, Shimotsuga, Tochigi, Japan
e-mail: umesawa@dokkyomed.ac.jp; genkoba@dokkyomed.ac.jp

K. Uchiyama
Department of Public Health, Dokkyo Medical University, Shimotsuga, Tochigi, Japan

Laboratory of International Environmental Health, Center for International Cooperation, Dokkyo Medical University, Shimotsuga, Tochigi, Japan
e-mail: koji-u@dokkyomed.ac.jp

H. Taneichi
Department of Orthopaedic Surgery, Dokkyo Medical University, Shimotsuga, Tochigi, Japan
e-mail: taneichi@dokkyomed.ac.jp

M. Washio, G. Kobashi (eds.), *Epidemiological Studies of Specified Rare and Intractable Disease*, Current Topics in Environmental Health and Preventive Medicine, https://doi.org/10.1007/978-981-13-1096-6_2

The concept of ankylosing spinal hyperostosis (ASH) was developed by Forestier in 1950 [1]. ASH is defined as the presence of bony outgrowths or hyperostoses, mainly in the dorsal region of the vertebrae. Hyperostoses arise from the anterolateral aspect of the vertebral bodies [1]. Tsukimoto reported a Japanese case of a syndrome of spinal cord compression due to the ossification of the "posterior" longitudinal ligament 10 years later [2].

In this section, we provide information about the risk factors for OPLL, including gene polymorphisms, as well as its epidemiology, etiology, and current clinical knowledge.

2.2 Epidemiology and Etiology of OPLL

2.2.1 Epidemiology

Table 2.1 shows the previously reported prevalence of OPLL [3–9]. The prevalence of OPLL in the Asian population is generally higher than in the Western population. Recently, computed tomography (CT)-based cross-sectional studies were conducted to evaluate OPLL [7–9]. The prevalence of cervical OPLL among Japanese who underwent positron emission tomography and CT (PET-CT) during health checkups was 8.3% in men and 3.4% in women [8], and those of thoracic OPLL was 1.4% in men and 2.0% in women. The prevalence of cervical OPLL among residents in the San Francisco area who underwent head and neck CT for trauma screening was 2.2% and it was higher in Asian Americans (4.8%) than in Caucasian Americans (1.3%), African Americans (2.1%), and Native Americans (3.2%) [7]. The prevalence of OPLL among Korean subjects was 5.7%, which is 8.8% in men and 4.2% in women [9]. This Korean study also reported that the prevalence of OPLL was higher in older subjects compared with younger subjects. The prevalence of OPLL in subjects aged 70 years or older was 16.9% in men and 8.9% in women, while they were 3.5% and 1.7% in subjects in their 30 s, respectively [9].

2.2.2 Etiology

Multiple causes of OPLL were reported. Currently, genetic factors seem to be important risk factors for OPLL, as seen in the results of Japanese family and twin studies [10, 11]. Today, many case–control studies and sibling-pair linkage studies are being conducted to detect genetic factors. We discuss individual associations between gene polymorphism and the risk of OPLL later in this review. Except for genetic factors, a few epidemiological studies examined the associations between the risk of OPLL with obesity, history of disease, and lifestyle factors using case–control designs. We also introduce the results of these studies and the results of cross-sectional studies conducted later on.

Table 2.1 Prevalence of ossification of the posterior longitudinal ligament (OPLL)

Nations	Number of subjects	Characteristics of subjects	Mean age of subjects	Definition	Prevalence	Reference number
Japan	1562 (524 male and 1038 female)	Japanese male and female residents	Men: 66.2 y.o. Women: 64.4 y.o.	X-ray	Men: 3.2% Women: 1.3%	[3]
Japan	4802	Japanese men, belonging to Self-Defense Force	51.4 y.o.	X-ray	4.1%	[4]
Taiwan	–	Taiwanese	–	–	2.8%	[5]
Singapore	5167	Patients who attended the Mount Elizabeth Hospital in Singapore for cervical spine complaints	–	–	0.8%	[6]
USA(San Francisco)	3161 (1593 Caucasians, 624 Asians, 472 Hispanics, 326 Africans, 62 native Americans and 84 others)	Patients who perceived head and neck CT for trauma screening	51.2 y.o.	CT	2.2%	[7]
Japan	1500 (888 male and 612 female)	Japanese subjects who perceived PETCT for their private health check	57 y.o.	PETCT	Men: 8.3% Women: 3.4%	[8]
Korea	3240 (1084 male and 2156 female)	Korean men and women, patients who underwent 3DCT	50.7 y.o.	3DCT	Men: 8.8% Women: 4.2%	[9]

y.o. years old, *CT* computed tomography, *PETCT* positron emission tomography–CT

2.3 Clinical Aspect of OPLL

2.3.1 Symptoms

The proportion of OPLL subjects who had symptoms was between 20 and 50% [12, 13]. Symptomatic OPLL causes myelopathy with or without radiculopathy, and symptoms such as hand clumsiness, gait disturbance, numbness of arms and legs, and pain in arms and back of the head and neck may be present. According to a nationwide survey in 1975, the proportion of OPLL subjects who showed mild to moderate disability of the upper extremities was 42.8% [12]. Due to dysfunctions of the lower extremities, 10.1% of OPLL subjects were nonambulatory and 12.9% were able to ambulate only with support [12]. Although difficulty of neck movements may occur, its frequency has not yet reported.

2.3.2 Evaluation and Diagnosis

OPLL may be detected by X-rays. CT scans allow the orthopedist to easily determine the type and expansion of OPLL. OPLL may be classified into four types according to ossification morphology. These types are the continuous type, wherein ossification is continuously spread for several segments; the segmental type, wherein ossification is separated but spread for several segments; the mixed type, wherein there is a mix of the continuous type and segmental type; and the localized type, wherein ossification is located on only one or two segments [Fig. 2.1]. In a Japanese study, the prevalence of continuous type, segmental type, mixed type, and localized type were 43.3%, 26.7%, 23.3%, and 6.7%, respectively [3]. A Korean study reported that the prevalence of continuous type, segmental type (multiple segmental type), mixed type, and localized type (single segmental type) were 8.6%, 37.3%, 11.4%, and 34.6%, respectively [9].

In Japan, the diagnostic criteria for OPLL are defined by orthopedists [13], and diagnosis is made when the following 2 criteria are met:

1. Ossification of the posterior longitudinal ligament as detected by X-ray or CT.
2. The presence of at least one of the following symptoms: cervical myelopathy caused by chronic spinal cord compression, radiculopathy, and dysfunction of cervical spine mobility caused by restriction of the joints' movable range.

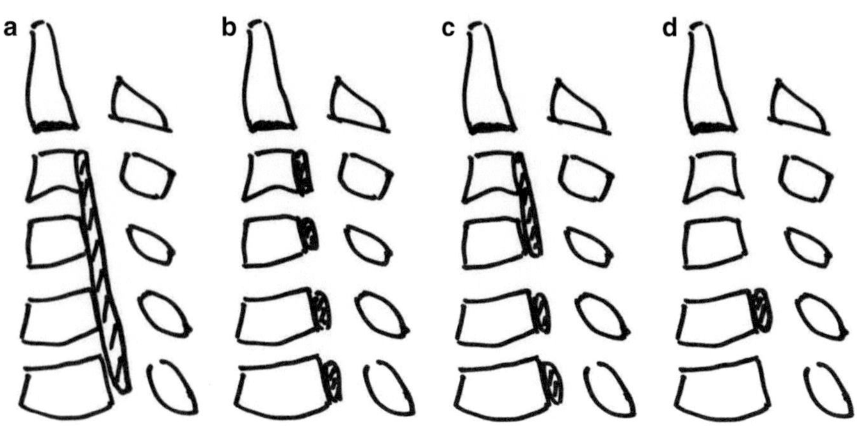

Fig. 2.1 Types of ossification of the posterior longitudinal ligament: (**a**) continuous type, (**b**) segmental type, (**c**) mixed type, and (**d**) localized type

2.3.3 Care

OPLL treatment strategies consist of conservative treatment and surgery. In Japan, OPLL care guidelines suggest that OPLL with symptoms of myelopathy or radiculomyelopathy should be surgically treated, while OPLL without these symptoms should be conservatively treated, including administration of medications. However, conservative treatment is backed by only a few solid evidences [13].

2.3.4 Prognosis

The natural history of OPLL is lengthy. A prospective study of Japanese OPLL patients revealed that 71% of patients without symptoms of myeloradiculopathy at the first orthopedic visit did not show any symptoms of myeloradiculopathy at follow-up examination 30 years later [14].

The effects of surgery have also been reported [13, 14]. Among patients who have walking difficulties that prevent them from full-time employment or the ability to do any housework but whose condition was not so severe as to require someone else's help to walk, 12% with Nurick grade 3 or more who were surgically treated suffered further deterioration because of myeloradiculopathy, while 89% of the patients were treated conservatively [14].

A Japanese study using data from 3 years' follow-up of 30 OPLL patients failed to find any risk factors significantly associated with OPLL prognosis [3].

2.4 Risk Factors for OPLL

2.4.1 Genetic Factors

Table 2.2 shows the reported genetic factors associated with OPLL [15–48]. Twenty-nine case–control studies reported 19 genes whose single nucleotide polymorphisms (SNPs) were associated with a higher risk of OPLL [15–18, 21, 22, 24, 26, 27, 29–33, 35–48]. A study of Chinese OPLL patients was conducted by targeted exome sequencing of the 11 OPLL-associated genes [19]. Another study of Chinese OPLL patients utilized whole exome sequencing (WES) and found a positive association between *PTCH1* and OPLL [30]. Two studies of Japanese OPLL patients which used genome-wide association studies (GWAS) to detect SNPs associated with OPLL found that 3 gene mutations and 5 intergenic DNA mutations were positively associated with OPLL [23, 49].

Table 2.2 Genes whose polymorphism is positively associated with the risk of ossification of the posterior longitudinal ligament (OPLL)

			Subjects			Reference
Genes		Location	Characteristics	Study design	Number (case vs. control)	Number
ACE	Angiotensin 1 converting enzyme	17q23.3	Korean	Case–control	95 vs. 274	[15]
BID	BH3 interacting domain death agonist	22q11.21	Korean	Case–control	157 vs. 209	[16]
BMP2	Bone morphogenic protein 2	20p 12.3	Chinese	Case–control	57 vs. 135	[17]
			Chinese	Case–control	420 vs. 506	[18]
			Chinese	NGS	55 (M:32, F:23) patients of OPLL	[19]
BMP4	Bone morphogenic protein 4	14q22.2	Japanese	Sibling study	126 sib-pair	[20]
			Chinese	Case–control	179 vs. 298	[21]
			Chinese	Case–control	450 vs. 550	[22]
CCDC91	Coiled-coil domain containing 91	12p11.22	Japanese	GWAS	1660(1112 + 548) vs. 13,279(6810 + 6469)	[23]
COL11A2	Collagen 11A2	6p21.32	Japanese	Case–control	18 vs. 51	[24]
			Japanese	Sibling study	91 sib-pair	[25]
			Japanese	Case–control	195 vs. 187	[26]
			Japanese	Case–control	161 vs. 163	[27]
			Chinese	NGS	55 (M:32, F:23) patients of OPLL	[19]
COL6A1	Collagen 6A1	21 q22.3	Japanese	Sibling study	142 sib-pair	[28]
			Chinese	Case–control	122(OPLL:90, OPLL+OLF:32) vs. 155	[29]
			Chinese	NGS	55 (M:32, F:23) patients of OPLL	[19]
COL17A1	Collagen type XVII alpha 1 chain	10q25.1	Chinese	Case–control	28 vs. 100	[30]
ENPP1(NPP1)	Ectonucleotide pyrophosphatase phosphodiesterase 1	6q23.2	Japanese	Case–control	323 vs. 332	[31]
			Japanese	Case–control	180 vs. 265	[32]
			Chinese	Case–control	95 vs. 90	[33]
			Japanese	Case report	1	[34]

ESR1	Estrogen receptor	6q25.1–q25.2	Japanese women	Case–control	120 vs. 306	[35]
FGFR1	FGF receptor 1	8p11.23	Korean	Case–control	157 vs. 222	[36]
			Chinese	NGS	55 (M:32, F:23) patients of OPLL	[19]
GDF2(BMP9)	Growth differentiation factor 2 (bone morphogenetic protein 9)	10q11.22	Chinese	Case–control	450 vs. 550	[37]
IFNG	Interferon gamma	12q15	Korean	Case–control	135 vs. 222	[38]
IL15RA	Interleukin 15 receptor alpha	10p15.1	Korean	Case–control	166 vs. 230	[39]
			Chinese	Case–control	235 vs. 250	[40]
IL1B	Interleukin 1 beta	2q14.1	Japanese women	Case–control	120 vs. 306	[35]
LOC100506393	(uncharacterized)	12p12.2	Japanese	GWAS	1660(112 + 548) vs. 13,279(6810 + 6469)	[23]
PTCH1	Protein patched homolog 1	9q22.32	Chinese	WES (in case–control)	2 females (in 28 vs. 100)	[30]
RSPO2	Roof plate-specific spondin-2	8q23.1	Japanese	GWAS	1660(112 + 548) vs. 13,279(6810 + 6469)	[23]
RUNX2	Runt-related transcription factor 2	6p21.1	Chinese	Case–control	82 vs. 118	[41]
			Chinese	Case–control	80 vs. 80	[42]
RXRB	Retinoic X receptor beta	6p21.3	Japanese	Case–control	134 vs. 158	[43]
TGFB1	Transforming growth factor beta 1	19q13.2	Japanese	Case–control	46 vs. 319	[44]
TGFB3	Transforming growth factor beta 3	14q24.3	Japanese	Case–control	711 vs. 896	[45]
TGFBR2	Transforming growth factor beta receptor 2	3p24.1	Korean	Case–control	21 vs. 42	[46]
VDR	Vitamin D receptor	12q13.11	Japanese	Case–control	63 vs. 126	[47]
VKORC1	Vitamin K epoxide reductase complex subunit 1	16p11.2	Korean	Case–control	98 vs. 200	[48]

GWAS genome-wide association study, *NGS* next-generation sequencing, *WES* whole exome sequencing

Specifically, the following genetic factors were associated with the risk of OPLL: angiotensin 1 converting enzyme gene (*ACE*), BH3 interacting domain death agonist gene (*BID*), bone morphogenic protein 2 gene (*BMP2*), bone morphogenic protein 4 gene (*BMP4*), coiled-coil domain containing 91 gene (*CCDC91*), collagen 6A1 gene (*COL6A1*), collagen 11A2 gene (*COL11A2*), collagen type XVII alpha 1 chain gene (*COL17A1*), ectonucleotide pyrophosphatase phosphodiesterase 1 gene (*ENPP1*), estrogen receptor gene (ESR1), FGF receptor 1 gene (FGFR1), growth differentiation factor 2 gene (bone morphogenetic protein 9 gene) (*GDF2* (*BMP9*)), interferon gamma gene (*IFNG*), interleukin 1 beta gene (*IL1B*), interleukin 15 receptor alpha gene (*IL15RA*), *LOC100506393* which was not characterized, protein patched homolog 1 gene (*PTCH1*), roof plate-specific spondin-2 gene (*RSPO2*), runt-related transcription factor 2 gene (*RUNX2*), retinoic X receptor beta gene (*RXRB*), transforming growth factor beta 1 gene (*TGFB1*), transforming growth factor beta 3 gene (*TGFB3*), transforming growth factor beta receptor 2 gene (*TGFBR2*), vitamin D receptor gene (*VDR*), and vitamin K epoxide reductase complex subunit 1 gene (*VKORC1*).

On the other hand, several genetic factors we listed as follows were tested and failed to find the associations with OPLL in other studies: *BMP2, BMP4, COL6A1, COL11A2, ENPP1, ESR1, GDF2(BMP9), TGFB1, TGFBR2,* and *VDR* [19, 20, 24, 35, 41, 45, 50–54].

BMP2 mutation was reported to be positively associated with OPLL in 2 case–control Chinese studies and in 1 targeted exome sequencing Chinese study [17–19], while case–control studies of Japanese, Chinese, and Korean showed no association between *BMP2* OPLL [24, 41, 50]. *BMP4* mutation was reported to have a positive association with OPLL in a Japanese sibling study and in 2 case–control Chinese studies [20–22], however, a Chinese targeted exome sequencing study found no association between them [19]. The positive association between *COL6A1* mutation and the risk of OPLL was reported by a Chinese case–control study, a Japanese sibling study, and a Chinese targeted exome sequencing study [19, 28, 29], while case–control studies of Chinese and Koreans did not show significant association between them [41, 50]. *COLL11A2* mutation was reported to have a positive association with OPLL in 3 Japanese case–control studies, a Japanese sibling study, and a Chinese targeted exome sequencing study [19, 24–27], while a Japanese case–control study did not show significant associations between them [45]. *ENPP1* mutation was positively associated with the risk of OPLL in Chinese and Japanese case–control studies [31–33], while 2 case–control Japanese studies and a Japanese sibling study did not find significant associations between them [20, 45, 51]. The association between *ESR1* mutation and the risk of OPLL in Japanese women was reported [35], however, a Chinese targeted exome sequencing study did not show any significant associations between them [19]. *GDF2(BMP9)* mutation was reported to have a positive association with the risk of OPLL in Chinese individuals [37], however, a Chinese targeted exome sequencing study did not show significant associations between them [19]. *TGFB1* mutation was reportedly associated with the risk of OPLL in a Japanese case–control study [44], however, the same association was not found in 2 Japanese case–control studies, a Korean case–control study, and a Chinese targeted exome sequencing study [19, 45, 52, 53]. *TGFBR2* mutation was also reportedly associated with the risk for OPLL in a Korean case–control study [46], while the same association was not found in a Chinese targeted exome sequencing study [19]. The association between *VDR* mutation and the risk for OPLL was reported in a Japanese case–control study [47], while the association was not significant in another Japanese case–control study and a Chinese case–control study [35, 41].

In addition to the genetic factors shown above, *ENPP4, LEPR,* and *TLR5* were examined for their association with the risk for OPLL, however, there were no associations between them [19, 50, 54].

2.4.2 Nongenetic Factors

Table 2.3 shows the risk factors previously reported for OPLL, except for genetic factors. These reports involved Asian subjects.

Higher body mass index (BMI) was positively associated with the risk of OPLL. According to a univariate analysis in a case–control Japanese study [55], subjects who were overweight, with BMI $\geq$ 25 kg/m^2, and aged 40 years and above had 4.11 times higher OPLL risk compared with subjects who were lighter and younger. In addition, subjects whose maximum BMI before manifestation was $\geq$25 kg/m^2 showed 3.52 times higher OPLL risk compared with subjects who were lighter. In a multivariate analysis, subjects whose maximum BMI before manifestation was $\geq$25 kg/m^2 showed 3.49 times higher risk for OPLL compared with subjects who had a lower BMI. However, the association between being overweight, age greater than 40, and the risk for OPLL was not significant. The authors also examined the differences of BMI between OPLL subjects and control subjects at age 20 years and 40 years and found that BMI at age 40 years was higher in OPLL subjects than in control subjects, while they did not find significant differences in BMI at age 20 years [55].

A cross-sectional Japanese study reported on a history of diabetes mellitus and showed a positive association between glucose intolerance and prevalence of OPLL [4]. A case–control Japanese study also reported that a history of diabetes mellitus was positively associated with the risk for OPLL [55]. In a multivariate analysis, subjects who had a history of diabetes mellitus showed 11.78 times higher risk of OPLL compared with subjects who did not have diabetes. This study also reported that a history of lumbago was positively associated with the risk for OPLL. Subjects who had a history of low back pain showed 4.07 times higher risk for OPLL compared with subjects who did not. In addition, this study reported that a history of whiplash injury and a natural lack of body pliability are positively associated with the risk for OPLL in univariate analysis. However, the association was not significant after adjusting for other risk factors. As for history of illness, a family history of myocardial infarction was positively associated with the risk for OPLL in a Japanese study [47]. On the other hand, a case–control Korean study showed no significant associations between hypertension or diabetes mellitus and the risk for

Table 2.3 Risk factors associated with the risk of ossification of the posterior longitudinal ligament (OPLL)

Risk factors	Subjects			Association with the risk of OPLL	Reference number
	Characteristic	Study design	Number		
Age	Korean	Cross-sectional	185 cases in 3240 subjects	Positive	[9]
Higher height	Japanese	Cross-sectional	30 cases in 1562 subjects	Positive	[3]
Higher body weight	Japanese	Cross-sectional	30 cases in 1562 subjects	Positive	[3]
BMI ≥25 at examination	Japanese	Cross-sectional	198 cases in 4802 subjects	Positive	[4]
BMI at 40 yo.	Japanese	Case–control	69 cases vs. 138 controls	Positive	[55]
BMI ≥25 before manifestation	Japanese	Case–control	69 cases vs. 138 controls	Positive	[55]
Family history of MI	Japanese	Case–control	63 cases vs. 126 controls	Positive	[47]
History of DM	Japanese	Case–control	69 cases vs. 138 controls	Positive	[55]
History of lumbago	Japanese	Case–control	69 cases vs. 138 controls	Positive	[55]
Glucose intolerance	Japanese	Cross-sectional	198 cases in 4802 subjects	Positive	[4]
Serum levels of pentosidine	Japanese	Cross-sectional	30 cases in 1562 subjects	Positive	[3]
Long working hours (≥80 h/week)	Japanese	Case–control	63 cases vs. 126 controls	Positive	[47]
Night shift worker	Japanese	Case–control	63 cases vs. 126 controls	Positive	[47]
Moderate sleep time (6–8 h/day)	Japanese	Case–control	69 cases vs. 138 controls	Negative	[56]
Regular sleep habit	Japanese	Case–control	69 cases vs. 138 controls	Negative	[56]
Salted products intake (pickles)	Japanese	Case–control	69 cases vs. 138 controls	Positive	[57]
High salt diet intake	Taiwanese	Case–control	98 cases vs. 98 controls	Positive	[58]
Daily rice intake	Japanese	Case–control	69 cases vs. 138 controls	Negative	[57]
Daily meat intake	Taiwanese	Case–control	98 cases vs. 98 controls	Negative	[58]
Chicken intake	Japanese	Case–control	69 cases vs. 138 controls	Negative	[57]

Table 2.3 (continued)

	Subjects			Association with the risk of OPLL	Reference number
Risk factors	Characteristic	Study design	Number		
Soyfood intake	Japanese	Case–control	69 cases vs. 138 controls	Negative	[57]
BMD of the lumbar spine	Japanese	Cross-sectional	30 cases in 1562 subjects	Positive	[3]
BMD of the femoral neck	Japanese	Cross-sectional	30 cases in 1562 subjects	Positive	[3]

BMD bone mineral density, *BMI* body mass index, *DM* diabetes mellitus, *MI* myocardial infarction

OPLL [48]. A Taiwanese case–control study also showed no association between plasma sugar levels and the risk of OPLL [58].

The associations between lifestyle-related factors and the risk of OPLL were reported in Japanese case–control studies [55–57] and a Taiwanese case–control study [58].

Rice is a staple in the Japanese diet and subjects with non-daily intakes of rice, in the period of 5 years before the survey, showed 3.0 times higher risk for OPLL compared with subjects who ate rice daily [57]. Subjects in Japan who ate salted products equal to or more than four times per week in the period of 5 years before survey also showed 1.6 times higher risk for OPLL compared with subjects who did not. On the other hand, a Japanese study showed that frequent chicken and soyfood intake equal to or more than three times per week in the period of 5 years before the survey showed a negative association with the risk for OPLL. Subjects who frequently ate chicken showed 0.5 times lower risk of OPLL compared with subjects who did not. Subjects who frequently ate soyfood showed 0.4 times lower risk for OPLL compared with subjects who did not. In a Taiwanese study, high salt intake and low meat intake were positively associated with the risk for OPLL [58]. In the study, OPLL patients tended to prefer high salt diets and pickled foods and did not consume meat on a daily basis.

In terms of working conditions, working hours of more than 80 h per week and working a night shift were positively associated with the risk for OPLL [47]. Subjects who worked more than 80 h per week showed 8.77 times higher risk for OPLL compared with subjects who did not and subjects who worked a night shift showed 2.92 times higher risk for OPLL compared with subjects who did not.

Subjects who had 5 h or less of sleep per day showed 6.64 times higher risk for OPLL compared with subjects who had 6 to 8 h of sleep per day [56]. In addition, subjects who had regular sleeping habits showed 0.44 times lower risk for OPLL compared with subjects who did not.

In addition, moderate exercise at least once a week was not associated with the risk for OPLL [56]. Current smoking and drinking habits at least once per week did not show an association with the risk for OPLL [56].

In Japan, the associations between serum biomarkers and risk of OPLL were also examined. Two Japanese case–control studies showed a positive association between high serum leptin and risk for OPLL/ossification of spinal ligaments (OSL) [59, 60]. Recently, a Japanese case–control study reported that serum high-sensitivity C-reactive protein (hs-CRP) was higher in subjects with OPLL than in subjects without OPLL [61].

2.5 Comments

We reviewed the risk factors for OPLL. Many risk factors are associated with OPLL manifestation and its progression. Genetic factors were examined, while lifestyle-related factors were not. Recently, studies were conducted on the associations between serum biomarkers and the risk of OPLL. Further studies that examine the associations between lifestyle-related factors and/or biomarkers and the risk for OPLL should be carried out in the future.

Generally, the risk factors for OPLL are divided into two categories, which are genetic factors and others. In the present article, we tried to interpret studies according to different aspects of risk factors, although the evidence was limited. We assumed that the risk factors of OPLL reported previously are as follows: structural factors, mechanical stimulation factors, inflammatory factors, and the others.

Structural factors consist of genes that influence body structure, such as *BMPs, COLs,* and *TGFBs*, and nutritional factors. Adequate body structure may be resistant to OPLL. Suggested mechanisms of diffuse idiopathic skeletal hyperostosis (DISH), which consist of entheseal calcification and ossification, were based on several pathways and are closely associated, and sometimes complicates, OPLL [3, 62–64]. We found several factors reported to be the associated with the risk for OPLL, such as *BMP2, COL6A1,* and insulin [65]. These risk factors may play the same roles for OPLL manifestation. As nutritional factors, the national dietary Japanese survey revealed that chicken and soy are major sources of protein intake in Japan [66]. In addition, infrequent rice intake may be associated with a lower intake of plant protein and Japanese adults consume almost 13% (8 g) of carbohydrates from rice per day [66].

Mechanical stimulation factors consist of excess body weight, history of lumbago, hard work, and inadequate sleep. Excess body weight may apply excessive loads to the spine and joints. Lumbago seems to be a result of excessively strenuous activities, which impacts the lower back. Hard work involves excessive work. Short sleeping times and irregular sleeping habits were positively associated with the risk of OPLL. We interpreted that insufficient recovery from daily fatigue may be associated with OPLL risk. Aside from this, excessive mechanical stimulation may cause inflammatory responses.

Inflammatory factors consist of genes that play roles in inflammatory mechanisms, such as ILs, and serum biomarkers, such as leptin and hs-CRP. Inflammation may increase the occurrence and hasten the progression of OPLL [61]. A history of diabetes mellitus and higher BMI may be included in these factors because they usually are associated with inflammation in body [67].

The mechanisms of OPLL are still unclear and there are many unresolved questions. Thus, we cannot determine which among the factors mentioned above is mainly related to the onset of OPLL. However, future research endeavors should clarify the mechanisms associated with OPLL, which are composed of some possible pathogenetic pathways in which respective genetic and nongenetic factors interact. Furthermore, future studies can also propose novel treatment strategies using both genetic and nongenetic factors to prevent OPLL.

References

1. Forestier J, Rotes-querol J. Senile ankylosing hyperostosis of the spine. Ann Rheum Dis. 1950;9:321–30.
2. Tsukimoto H. A case report: autopsy of syndrome of compression of spinal cord owing to ossification within spinal canal of cervical spines. Nippon Geka Hokan 29, 1003–1007 (in Japanese).
3. Yoshimura N, Nagata K, Muraki S, Oka H, Yoshida M, Enyo Y, et al. Prevalence and progression of radiographic ossification of the posterior longitudinal ligament and associated factors in the Japanese population: a 3-year follow-up of the ROAD study. Osteoporos Int. 2014;25:1089–98. https://doi.org/10.1007/s00198-013-2489-0.
4. Shingyouchi Y, Nagahama A, Niida M. Ligamentous ossification of the cervical spine in the late middle-aged Japanese men. Its relation to body mass index and glucose metabolism. Spine (Phila Pa 1976). 1996;21:2474–8.
5. Wang PN, Chen SS, Liu HC, Fuh JL, Kuo BI, Wang SJ. Ossification of the posterior longitudinal ligament of the spine. A case-control risk factor study. Spine (Phila Pa 1976). 1999;24:142–4.
6. Lee T, Chacha PB, Khoo J. Ossification of posterior longitudinal ligament of the cervical spine in non-Japanese Asians. Surg Neurol. 1991;35:40–4.
7. Fujimori T, Le H, Hu SS, Chin C, Pekmezci M, Schairer W, et al. Ossification of the posterior longitudinal ligament of the cervical spine in 3161 patients: a CT-based study. Spine (Phila Pa 1976). 2015;40:E394–403. https://doi.org/10.1097/BRS.0000000000000791.
8. Fujimori T, Watabe T, Iwamoto Y, Hamada S, Iwasaki M, Oda T. Prevalence, concomitance, and distribution of ossification of the spinal ligaments: results of whole spine CT scans in 1500 Japanese patients. Spine (Phila Pa 1976) 2016;41:1668–1676.
9. Sohn S, Chung CK, Yun TJ, Sohn CH. Epidemiological survey of ossification of the posterior longitudinal ligament in an adult Korean population: three-dimensional computed tomographic observation of 3,240 cases. Calcif Tissue Int. 2014;94:613–20.
10. Terayama K. Genetic studies on ossification of the posterior longitudinal ligament of the spine. Spine (Phila Pa 1976). 1989;14:1184–91.
11. Taketomi E, Sakou T, Matsunaga S, Yamaguchi M. Family study of a twin with ossification of the posterior longitudinal ligament in the cervical spine. Spine (Phila Pa 1976). 1992;17:S55–6.
12. Tsuyama N. Ossification of the posterior longitudinal ligament of the spine. Ossification of the posterior longitudinal ligament of the spine. Clin Orthop Relat Res. 1984;184:71-84.
13. The Japanese Orthopaedic Association. Japanese Orthopaedic Assciation (JOA) clinical practice guideline on the management of ossification of posterior longitudinal ligament of the cervical spine, 2011. Tokyo: Nankodo Co. 2011. p. 75.

14. Matsunaga S, Sakou T, Taketomi E, Komiya S. Clinical course of patients with ossification of the posterior longitudinal ligament: a minimum 10-year cohort study. J Neurosurg. 2004;100(3 Suppl Spine):245–8.
15. Kim DH, Yun DH, Kim HS, Min SK, Yoo SD, Lee KH, et al. The insertion/deletion polymorphism of angiotensin I converting enzyme gene is associated with ossification of the posterior longitudinal ligament in the Korean population. Ann Rehabil Med. 2014;38:1–5. https://doi.org/10.5535/arm.2014.38.1.1.
16. Chon J, Hong JH, Kim J, Han YJ, Lee BW, Kim SC, et al. Association between BH3 interacting domain death agonist (BID) gene polymorphism and ossification of the posterior longitudinal ligament in Korean population. Mol Biol Rep. 2014;41:895–9. https://doi.org/10.1007/s11033-013-2933-4.
17. Wang H, Liu D, Yang Z, Tian B, Li J, Meng X, et al. Association of bone morphogenetic protein-2 gene polymorphisms with susceptibility to ossification of the posterior longitudinal ligament of the spine and its severity in Chinese patients. Eur Spine J. 2008 Jul;17(7):956–64. https://doi.org/10.1007/s00586-008-0651-8.
18. Yan L, Chang Z, Liu Y, Li YB, He BR, Hao DJ. A single nucleotide polymorphism in the human bone morphogenetic protein-2 gene (109T > G) affects the Smad signaling pathway and the predisposition to ossification of the posterior longitudinal ligament of the spine. Chin Med J (Engl). 2013;126:1112-8.
19. Chen X, Guo J, Cai T, Zhang F, Pan S, Zhang L, et al. Targeted next-generation sequencing reveals multiple deleterious variants in OPLL-associated genes. Sci Rep. 2016;6:26962. https://doi.org/10.1038/srep26962.
20. Furushima K, Shimo-Onoda K, Maeda S, Nobukuni T, Ikari K, Koga H, et al. Large-scale screening for candidate genes of ossification of the posterior longitudinal ligament of the spine. J Bone Miner Res. 2002;17:128–37.
21. Meng XL, Wang H, Yang H, Hai Y, Tian BP, Lin X. T allele at site 6007 of bone morphogenetic protein-4 gene increases genetic susceptibility to ossification of the posterior longitudinal ligament in male Chinese Han population. Chin Med J (Engl). 2010;123:2537-42.
22. Ren Y, Feng J, Liu ZZ, Wan H, Li JH, Lin X. A new haplotype in BMP4 implicated in ossification of the posterior longitudinal ligament (OPLL) in a Chinese population. J Orthop Res. 2012;30:748–56. https://doi.org/10.1002/jor.21586.
23. Nakajima M, Takahashi A, Tsuji T, Karasugi T, Baba H, Uchida K, et al. A genome-wide association study identifies susceptibility loci for ossification of the posterior longitudinal ligament of the spine. Nat Genet. 2014;46:1012–6. https://doi.org/10.1038/ng.3045.
24. Koga H, Hayashi K, Taketomi E, Matsunaga S, Yashiki S, Fujiyoshi T, et al. Restriction fragment length polymorphism of genes of the alpha 2(XI) collagen, bone morphogenetic protein-2, alkaline phosphatase, and tumor necrosis factor-alpha among patients with ossification of posterior longitudinal ligament and controls from the Japanese population. Spine (Phila Pa 1976). 1996;21:469–73.
25. Koga H, Sakou T, Taketomi E, Hayashi K, Numasawa T, Harata S. Yet al. Leppert M. Genetic mapping of ossification of the posterior longitudinal ligament of the spine. Am J Hum Genet. 1998;62:1460–7.
26. Maeda S, Ishidou Y, Koga H, Taketomi E, Ikari K, Komiya S, et al. Functional impact of human collagen alpha2(XI) gene polymorphism in pathogenesis of ossification of the posterior longitudinal ligament of the spine. J Bone Miner Res. 2001;16:948–57.
27. Maeda S, Koga H, Matsunaga S, Numasawa T, Ikari K, Furushima K, et al. Gender-specific haplotype association of collagen alpha2 (XI) gene in ossification of the posterior longitudinal ligament of the spine. J Hum Genet. 2001;46:1–4.
28. Tanaka T, Ikari K, Furushima K, Okada A, Tanaka H, Furukawa K, et al. Genomewide linkage and linkage disequilibrium analyses identify COL6A1, on chromosome 21, as the locus for ossification of the posterior longitudinal ligament of the spine. Am J Hum Genet. 2003;73:812–22.

29. Kong Q, Ma X, Li F, Guo Z, Qi Q, Li W, et al. COL6A1 polymorphisms associated with ossification of the ligamentum flavum and ossification of the posterior longitudinal ligament. Spine (PhilaPa1976). 2007;32:2834–8. https://doi.org/10.1097/BRS.0b013e31815b761c.
30. Wei W, He HL, Chen CY, Zhao Y, Jiang HL, Liu WT, et al. Whole exome sequencing implicates PTCH1 and COL17A1 genes in ossification of the posterior longitudinal ligament of the cervical spine in Chinese patients. Genet Mol Res. 2014;13:1794–804. https://doi.org/10.4238/2014.March.17.7.
31. Nakamura I, Ikegawa S, Okawa A, Okuda S, Koshizuka Y, Kawaguchi H, et al. Association of the human NPPS gene with ossification of the posterior longitudinal ligament of the spine (OPLL). Hum Genet. 1999;104:492–7.
32. Koshizuka Y, Kawaguchi H, Ogata N, Ikeda T, Mabuchi A, Seichi A, et al. Nucleotide pyrophosphatase gene polymorphism associated with ossification of the posterior longitudinal ligament of the spine. J Bone Miner Res. 2002;17:138–44.
33. He Z, Zhu H, Ding L, Xiao H, Chen D, Xue F. Association of NPP1 polymorphism with postoperative progression of ossification of the posterior longitudinal ligament in Chinese patients. Genet Mol Res. 2013;12:4648–55. https://doi.org/10.4238/2013.October.18.3.
34. Saito T, Shimizu Y, Hori M, Taguchi M, Igarashi T, Fukumoto S, et al. Patient with hypophosphatemic rickets and ossification of posterior longitudinal ligament caused by a novel homozygous mutation in ENPP1 gene. Bone. 2011;49:913–6. https://doi.org/10.1016/j.bone.2011.06.029.
35. Ogata N, Koshizuka Y, Miura T, Iwasaki M, Hosoi T, Shiraki M, et al. Association of bone metabolism regulatory factor gene polymorphisms with susceptibility to ossification of the posterior longitudinal ligament of the spine and its severity. Spine (Phila Pa 1976). 2002;27:1765–71.
36. Jun JK, Kim SM. Association study of fibroblast growth factor 2 and fibroblast growth factor receptors gene polymorphism in korean ossification of the posterior longitudinal ligament patients. J Korean Neurosurg Soc. 2012;52:7–13.
37. Ren Y, Liu ZZ, Feng J, Wan H, Li JH, Wang H, et al. Association of a BMP9 haplotype with ossification of the posterior longitudinal ligament (OPLL) in a Chinese population. PLoS One. 2012;7:e40587. https://doi.org/10.1371/journal.pone.0040587.
38. Kim KT, Kim DH, Chung JY, Lee S, Joo J, Nah SS, et al. Association of interferon gamma polymorphism with ossification of the posterior longitudinal ligament in the korean population. Immunol Investig. 2012;41:876–87. https://doi.org/10.3109/08820139.2012.714437.
39. Kim DH, Jeong YS, Chon J, Yoo SD, Kim HS, Kang SW, Chung JH, Kim KT, Cytokine YDH. Association between interleukin 15 receptor, alpha (IL15RA) polymorphism and Korean patients with ossification of the posterior longitudinal ligament. Cytokine. 2011;55:343–6. https://doi.org/10.1016/j.cyto.2011.05.016.
40. Guo Q, Lv SZ, Wu SW, Tian X, Li ZY. Association between single nucleotide polymorphism of IL15RA gene with susceptibility to ossification of the posterior longitudinal ligament of the spine. J Orthop Surg Res. 2014;9:103. https://doi.org/10.1186/s13018-014-0103-6.
41. Liu Y, Zhao Y, Chen Y, Shi G, Yuan W. RUNX2 polymorphisms associated with OPLL and OLF in the Han population. Clin Orthop Relat Res. 2010;468:3333–41. https://doi.org/10.1007/s11999-010-1511-5.
42. Chang F, Li L, Gao G, Ding S, Yang J, Zhang T, et al. Role of Runx2 polymorphisms in risk and prognosis of ossification of posterior longitudinal ligament. J Clin Lab Anal. 31. doi: https://doi.org/10.1002/jcla.22068.
43. Numasawa T, Koga H, Ueyama K, Maeda S, Sakou T, Harata S, et al. Human retinoic X receptor beta: complete genomic sequence and mutation search for ossification of posterior longitudinal ligament of the spine. J Bone Miner Res. 1999;14:500–8.
44. Kamiya M, Harada A, Mizuno M, Iwata H, Yamada Y. Association between a polymorphism of the transforming growth factor-beta1 gene and genetic susceptibility to ossification of the posterior longitudinal ligament in Japanese patients. Spine (Phila Pa 1976). 2001;26:1264–6.

45. Horikoshi T, Maeda K, Kawaguchi Y, Chiba K, Mori K, Koshizuka Y, et al. A large-scale genetic association study of ossification of the posterior longitudinal ligament of the spine. Hum Genet. 2006;119:611–6.
46. Jekarl DW, Paek CM, An YJ, Kim YJ, Kim M, Kim Y, et al. TGFBR2 gene polymorphism is associated with ossification of the posterior longitudinal ligament. J Clin Neurosci. 2013;20:453–6. https://doi.org/10.1016/j.jocn.2012.05.031.
47. Kobashi G, Ohta K, Washio M, Okamoto K, Sasaki S, Yokoyama T, et al. FokI variant of vitamin D receptor gene and factors related to atherosclerosis associated with ossification of the posterior longitudinal ligament of the spine: a multi-hospital case-control study. Spine (Phila Pa 1976). 2008;33:E553–8. https://doi.org/10.1097/BRS.0b013e31817e9de2.
48. Chin DK, Han IB, Ropper AE, Jeon YJ, Kim DH, Kim YS, et al. Association of VKORC1-1639G>A polymorphism with susceptibility to ossification of the posterior longitudinal ligament of the spine: a Korean study. Acta Neurochir. 2013;155:1937–42. https://doi.org/10.1007/s00701-013-1747-4.
49. Karasugi T, Nakajima M, Ikari K. Genetic study Group of Investigation Committee on ossification of the spinal ligaments. A genome-wide sib-pair linkage analysis of ossification of the posterior longitudinal ligament of the spine. J Bone Miner Metab. 2013;31:136–43. https://doi.org/10.1007/s00774-012-0404-y.
50. Kim KH, Kuh SU, Park JY, Lee SJ, Park HS, Chin DK, et al. Association between BMP-2 and COL6A1 gene polymorphisms with susceptibility to ossification of the posterior longitudinal ligament of the cervical spine in Korean patients and family members. Genet Mol Res. 2014;13:2240–7. https://doi.org/10.4238/2014.March.31.4.
51. Tahara M, Aiba A, Yamazaki M, Ikeda Y, Goto S, Moriya H, et al. The extent of ossification of posterior longitudinal ligament of the spine associated with nucleotide pyrophosphatase gene and leptin receptor gene polymorphisms. Spine (Phila Pa 1976). 2005;30:877–80.
52. Kawaguchi Y, Furushima K, Sugimori K, Inoue I, Kimura T. Association between polymorphism of the transforming growth factor-beta1 gene with the radiologic characteristic and ossification of the posterior longitudinal ligament. Spine (Phila Pa 1976). 2003;28:1424–6.
53. Han IB, Ropper AE, Jeon YJ, Park HS, Shin DA, Teng YD, et al. Association of transforming growth factor-beta 1 gene polymorphism with genetic susceptibility to ossification of the posterior longitudinal ligament in Korean patients. Genet Mol Res. 2013;12:4807–16. https://doi.org/10.4238/2013.February.28.26.
54. Chung WS, Nam DH, Jo DJ, Lee JH. Association of toll-like receptor 5 gene polymorphism with susceptibility to ossification of the posterior longitudinal ligament of the spine in korean population. J Korean Neurosurg Soc. 2011;49:8–12. https://doi.org/10.3340/jkns.2011.49.1.8.
55. Kobashi G, Washio M, Okamoto K, Sasaki S, Yokoyama T, Miyake Y, et al. High body mass index after age 20 and diabetes mellitus are independent risk factors for ossification of the posterior longitudinal ligament of the spine in Japanese subjects: a case-control study in multiple hospitals. Spine (Phila Pa 1976). 2004;29:1006–10.
56. Washio M, Kobashi G, Okamoto K, Sasaki S, Yokoyama T, Miyake Y, et al. Sleeping habit and other life styles in the prime of life and risk for ossification of the posterior longitudinal ligament of the spine (OPLL): a case-control study in Japan. J Epidemiol. 2004;14:168–73.
57. Okamoto K, Kobashi G, Washio M, Sasaki S, Yokoyama T, Miyake Y, et al. Dietary habits and risk of ossification of the posterior longitudinal ligaments of the spine (OPLL); findings from a case-control study in Japan. J Bone Miner Metab. 2004;22:612–7.
58. Wang PN, Chen SS, Liu HC, Fuh JL, Kuo BI, Wang SJ. Ossification of the posterior longitudinal ligament of the spine. A case-control risk factor study. Ossification of the posterior longitudinal ligament of the spine. A case-control risk factor study. Spine (Phila Pa 1976). 1999;24:142–4.
59. Shirakura Y, Sugiyama T, Tanaka H, Taguchi T, Kawai S. Hyperleptinemia in female patients with ossification of spinal ligaments. Biochem Biophys Res Commun. 2000;267:752–5.

60. Ikeda Y, Nakajima A, Aiba A, Koda M, Okawa A, Takahashi K, et al. Association between serum leptin and bone metabolic markers, and the development of heterotopic ossification of the spinal ligament in female patients with ossification of the posterior longitudinal ligament. Eur Spine J. 2011;20:1450–8. https://doi.org/10.1007/s00586-011-1688-7.
61. Kawaguchi Y, Nakano M, Yasuda T, Seki S, Suzuki K, Yahara Y, et al. Serum biomarkers in patients with ossification of the posterior longitudinal ligament (OPLL): inflammation in OPLL. PLoS One. 2017;12:e0174881. https://doi.org/10.1371/journal.pone.0174881.
62. McAfee PC, Regan JJ, Bohlman HH. Cervical cord compression from ossification of the posterior longitudinal ligament in non-orientals. J Bone Joint Surg Br. 1987;69:569–75.
63. Ehara S, Shimamura T, Nakamura R, Yamazaki K. Paravertebral ligamentous ossification: DISH, OPLL and OLF. Eur J Radiol. 1998;27:196–205.
64. Mader R, Verlaan JJ, Buskila D. Diffuse idiopathic skeletal hyperostosis: clinical features and pathogenic mechanisms. Nat Rev Rheumatol. 2013;9:741–50. https://doi.org/10.1038/nrrheum.2013.165.
65. Inamasu J, Guiot BH, Sachs DC. Ossification of the posterior longitudinal ligament: an update on its biology, epidemiology, and natural history. Neurosurgery. 2006;58:1027–39.
66. Ministry of Health, Labour and Welfare. [The National Health and Nutrition Survey in Japan, 2014] Tokyo, Japan (in Japanese).
67. Ebrahimi M, Heidari-Bakavoli AR, Shoeibi S, Mirhafez SR, Moohebati M, Esmaily H, et al. Association of serum hs-CRP levels with the presence of obesity, diabetes mellitus, and other cardiovascular risk factors. J Clin Lab Anal. 2016;30:672–6. https://doi.org/10.1002/jcla.21920.

Chapter 3
Descriptive and Analytic Epidemiology of Idiopathic Osteonecrosis of the Femoral Head in Japan

Wakaba Fukushima

Abstract Idiopathic osteonecrosis of the femoral head (ONFH) is a rare and multifactorial disease, which involves noninfectious and ischemic pathogenesis. ONFH has been designated as one of the targeted intractable diseases by the Ministry of Health, Labour and Welfare (MHLW) in Japan and its medical cost for treatment has been subsidized by public expenditure. Together with these policies, the epidemiology of ONFH in Japan has also been systematically elucidated by the Study Group on ONFH with academic support from the Study Group on Epidemiologic Research for Intractable Diseases (ERID), both of which are funded by the MHLW. This chapter summarizes the findings of descriptive and analytic epidemiology on ONFH which have been accumulated through collaborative efforts of the ONFH Study Group and the ERID Study Group. Methodologies in these epidemiologic studies include a nationwide epidemiologic survey and a hospital-based sentinel monitoring system to assess frequency and distribution of ONFH. Furthermore, case-control and cohort studies have been conducted to evaluate systemic steroid use and alcohol intake as two major risk factors for ONFH.

Keywords Osteonecrosis · Femoral head · Epidemiology · Steroid · Alcohol

3.1 Introduction

Idiopathic osteonecrosis of the femoral head (ONFH), also known as nontraumatic osteonecrosis or avascular osteonecrosis of the femoral head, is a rare and often progressive disease which typically involves noninfectious and ischemic pathogenesis. ONFH is considered to be a multifactorial disease and several potential mechanisms have been suggested including abnormal lipid or fat metabolism, nitric

W. Fukushima
Department of Public Health, Osaka City University Graduate School of Medicine, Osaka, Japan
e-mail: wakaba@med.osaka-cu.ac.jp

M. Washio, G. Kobashi (eds.), *Epidemiological Studies of Specified Rare and Intractable Disease*, Current Topics in Environmental Health and Preventive Medicine, https://doi.org/10.1007/978-981-13-1096-6_3

oxide-mediated apoptosis of osteoblasts and osteocytes, and thrombophilia or hypofibrinolysis [1–3]. The underlying etiology has not been fully elucidated, although some factors such as systemic steroid use and habitual alcohol consumption have been well known to be associated with ONFH development [1, 2]. Treatment options in the pre-collapse stage include osteotomy as a joint-preserving procedure, which is technically challenging because terminal blood flow in the femoral head is limited and biomechanical loads around the hip joint are complicated. Once collapse of the femoral head occurs, hip arthroplasty is needed and revision will be required in the future due to the survivorship of the artificial structures [3]. Eventually, bone destruction and loss of function in the hip joint substantially impair the patients' quality of life. In order to develop an appropriate strategy for disease prevention, treatment, and policy, it is fundamentally important to elucidate the epidemiology of ONFH in each country.

In Japan, the Ministry of Health and Welfare (later termed the Ministry of Health, Labour and Welfare [MHLW]) established a special program for "intractable diseases" in 1972. These are defined as rare diseases whose cause has not been determined and for which no specific medical treatment has been established. The program includes promoting research activities, eliminating patient co-payments for medical expenditures, and developing the necessary medical facilities. Under this program, the Study Group on Idiopathic Avascular Necrosis of the Femoral Head with support by a MHLW grant was launched in 1976. After 1982, this was re-named as "the Study Group on Idiopathic Osteonecrosis of the Femoral Head" (hereafter referred to as the ONFH Study Group). Later in 1992, ONFH was designated as one of the targeted intractable disease in Japan, and since then its medical costs have been subsidized by public expenditure [4].

Another study group funded by the MHLW, named "the Study Group on Epidemiologic Research for Intractable Diseases" (hereafter referred to as the ERID Study Group), was also launched in 1976 [5]. The ERID Study Group is comprised of epidemiologists and one of their missions is to provide academic support to other study groups on intractable diseases which are mainly comprised of clinicians. To date, the ONFH Study Group and the ERID Study Groups have cooperated with each other and a wide spectrum of epidemiologic studies has been employed. This chapter summarizes the main epidemiologic findings on ONFH in Japan from collaborative efforts of the two study groups, with the focus on two major risk factors for ONFH: systemic steroid use and habitual alcohol intake.

3.2 Descriptive Epidemiology (1): Nationwide Epidemiologic Survey

Since the mid-1990s, the prevalence of ONFH in Japan has been systematically clarified according to "a protocol for a nationwide epidemiologic survey on intractable diseases" as proposed by the ERID Study Group [6–9]. The procedure involves two stages: the first-stage survey, which estimates the number of patients visiting hospitals, and the second-stage survey, which reveals their demographic and clinical features. Nationwide epidemiologic surveys on ONFH have been conducted in 1995 [4, 10], 2005 [11], and 2015 [12]. It is noteworthy that the ONFH Study Group conducted nationwide epidemiologic surveys every 10 years from 1995 to 2015. Furthermore, using the same protocol in each survey enabled us to evaluate secular trends during the past two decades.

The targets in each survey were selected from all orthopedic departments in all hospitals in Japan by stratified random sampling according to inpatient bed numbers and hospital characteristics. Sampling fractions for each strata were as follows: 5% for general hospitals with 99 or fewer beds; 10% for 100 to 199 beds; 20% for 200 to 299 beds; 40% for 300 to 399 beds; 80% for 400 to 499 beds; 100% for 500 or more beds, university hospitals irrespective of the number of beds, and special departments where ONFH patients were likely to visit. The first-stage surveys were performed in January in 1995, 2005, and 2015, respectively, and the target departments were asked whether or not patients with ONFH visited their departments during the preceding 1 year (i.e., 1994, 2004, and 2014, respectively). The diagnostic criteria for ONFH, which had been proposed by the ONFH Study Group [13], was used with satisfying any two of the following five criteria: (1) collapse of the femoral head without joint space narrowing or acetabular abnormality on radiographs, including the crescent sign; (2) demarcating sclerosis in the femoral head without joint space narrowing or acetabular abnormality; (3) "cold in hot" on bone scans; (4) low-intensity band on T1-weighted magnetic resonance imaging (MRI), which was described as a "band-like pattern"; and (5) trabecular and marrow necrosis on histology. The sensitivity and specificity of the inclusion criteria were 91% and 99%, respectively, in comparison to histological diagnosis of ONFH as gold standard [14]. The estimated number of patients was initially calculated within each stratum according to the following formula: the estimated number of patients = the reported number of patients / (selection rate × response rate). Then, the estimated number of patients in each stratum was added to obtain the annual number of prevalent ONFH patients in Japan, and 95% confidence intervals (CI) were calculated with an assumption of multinominal hypergeometric distribution. The estimated annual prevalence of ONFH was further obtained using the total population of Japan as a denominator. Additionally, the estimated annual number of incident ONFH patients, which was defined as newly diagnosed ONFH patients during the year surveyed (i.e., 1994, 2004, and 2014, respectively), was calculated.

Table 3.1 shows the summary of the first-stage survey in three nationwide epidemiologic surveys. From 1994 to 2004, the estimated annual number of prevalent ONFH patients, the estimated annual prevalence of ONFH, and the estimated annual number of incident ONFH patients have increased approximately 1.5-fold (7400 patients to 11,400 patients, 5.9 per 100,000 population to 8.9 per 100,000 population, and 1500 patients to 2200 patients, respectively). Similarly, from 2004 to 2014, there was an approximate twofold increment in the estimated annual number of prevalent ONFH patients and the estimated annual prevalence of ONFH (11,400 patients to 23,100 patients, 8.9 per 100,000 population to 18.2 per 100,000 population, respectively). However, this was not observed for the estimated annual number

Table 3.1 Summary of the first-stage survey in three nationwide epidemiologic surveys of ONFH

Year conducted [reference No]	Year surveyed	Number of responding orthopedic departments (response rate, %)	Reported number of cases	Estimated annual number of prevalent cases during the year surveyed (95% CI)		Estimated annual prevalence during the year surveyed (per 100,000 population)	Estimated annual number of incident cases during the year surveyed[a] (95% CI)
1995 [4, 10]	1994	605 (57)	4271	7400	(6700–8200)	5.9	1500
2005 [11]	2004	577 (58)	5602	11,400	(10,100–12,800)	8.9	2200
2015 [12]	2014	738 (60)	13,563	23,100	(20,800–25,300)	18.2	2100

ONFH idiopathic osteonecrosis of the femoral head

[a]Defined as newly diagnosed ONFH cases during the year surveyed (i.e., 1994, 2004, and 2014, respectively)

of incident ONFH patients (2200 patients to 2100 patients). Explanations for this substantial increase in each figure from 1994 to 2004 could be that ONFH became a well-known disease in Japan after it was earmarked for financial support by the MHLW in 1992 and that diagnostic techniques advanced dramatically with the introduction of MRI. In contrast, possible reasons for the discrepancy between the increased number of prevalent cases and the stable number of incident cases during the most recent 10 years may be that ONFH is not a fatal disease in spite of frequent onset among those of middle-age, and therefore postoperative patients may have been accumulated over time. Nevertheless, the series of nationwide epidemiologic surveys clearly conveyed the disease burden of ONFH in Japan during the past two decades.

If target departments responded in the first-stage survey to report that they had a patient(s), they were invited to the second-stage survey to provide information on demographic and clinical characteristics for each patient using a structured questionnaire. Regarding the nationwide epidemiologic survey that was conducted in 2005, the second-stage survey gathered the information on 1502 ONFH patients, who were randomly sampled from the reported patients in the first-stage survey (i.e., prevalent cases who visited the target departments during 2004) [11]. The peak in the distribution of age at diagnosis was observed in those in their 40s among all subjects, in males in their 40s, and in females in their 30s (Fig. 3.1), which highlighted that ONFH frequently occurs in the middle-aged population. Table 3.2 shows the distribution of two major risk factors for ONFH patients: systemic steroid use and habitual alcohol intake. The proportion of each history was 51% for systemic steroid use, 31% for habitual alcohol intake, 3% for both steroid and alcohol

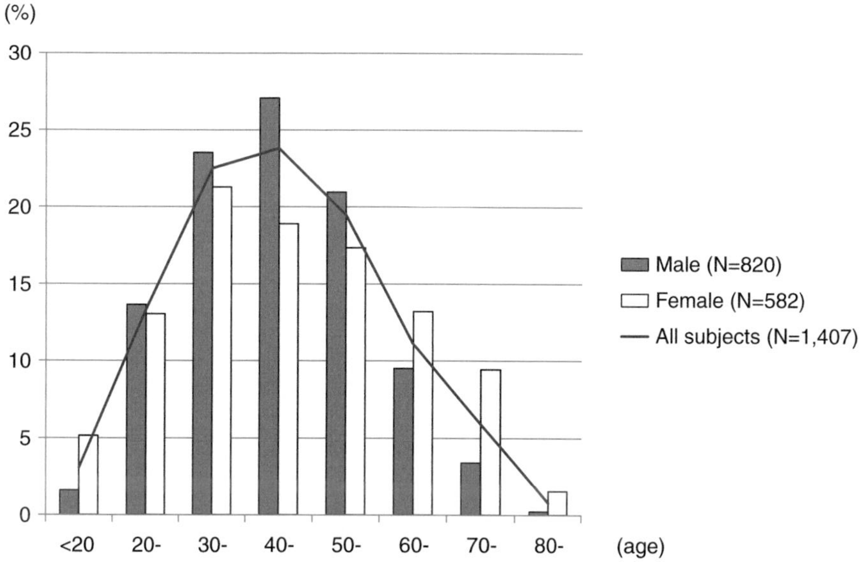

Fig. 3.1 Distribution of age at diagnosis is shown. Analysis is based on the subjects whose age at the time of diagnosis was available. There was no available information regarding gender for five subjects. [Source: Fukushima W, Fujioka M, Kubo T, Tamakoshi A, Nagai M, Hirota Y. Nationwide epidemiologic survey of idiopathic osteonecrosis of the femoral head. Clin Orthop Relat Res. 2010;468:2715–24]

Table 3.2 Distribution of potential causative factors among ONFH patients: a result from the second-stage survey in a nationwide epidemiologic survey in Japan, 2004

	All patients		Stratified by gender[a]				Stratified by age (years) at diagnosis[a]					
			Male		Female		<40		40–64		≥65	
	(n = 1502)		(n = 885)		(n = 612)		(n = 548)		(n = 706)		(n = 153)	
Variables	n (%)		n (%)		n (%)		n (%)		n (%)		n (%)	
Systemic steroid administration	760	(51)	295	(34)	462	(76)	325	(60)	340	(48)	58	(38)
Habitual alcohol use	456	(31)	415	(47)	39	(6)	146	(27)	253	(36)	26	(17)
Both	47	(3)	39	(4)	8	(1)	16	(3)	24	(3)	6	(4)
Neither	225	(15)	127	(15)	98	(16)	59	(11)	85	(12)	62	(41)
Unknown/not filled-in	14		9		5		2		4		1	

ONFH idiopathic osteonecrosis of the femoral head

Some totals of "%" do not equal 100% attributable to rounding

[a]There was no available information regarding gender for five patients and for age at diagnosis for 95 patients. [Source: Fukushima W, Fujioka M, Kubo T, Tamakoshi A, Nagai M, Hirota Y. Nationwide epidemiologic survey of idiopathic osteonecrosis of the femoral head. Clin Orthop Relat Res. 2010;468:2715–24]

intake, and 15% for neither steroid nor alcohol intake. Stratification by age at diagnosis revealed that there was a higher proportion of history of systemic steroid use in the younger age group (60% among those aged <40 years, 48% among those aged 40 to 64 years, and 38% among those aged ≥65 years). Among ONFH patients with history of systemic steroid use, systemic lupus erythematosus (SLE) was the most frequent underlying illness requiring steroid therapy (31%). Since SLE is characterized by early onset during the life course, these findings emphasized the importance of preventative strategies for ONFH among the younger population, including better steroid administration regimens for SLE.

3.3 Descriptive Epidemiology (2): A Hospital-Based Sentinel Monitoring System

A methodology for the nationwide epidemiologic survey on intractable diseases, which has been proposed by the ERID Study Group, is useful to understand the descriptive epidemiology in a specific country. However, it may not be the best method to evaluate secular trends of disease characteristics periodically due to significant effort and expensive costs. The ONFH Study Group therefore started a multicenter hospital-based sentinel monitoring system for ONFH (hereafter referred to as the ONFH sentinel monitoring system) in 1997 as an option to elucidate the descriptive epidemiology of ONFH. The monitoring system is currently ongoing and as of October 2017, a total of 35 hospitals from the ONFH Study Group are participating. The system is similar to the sentinel surveillance for infectious disease. The participating hospitals report the information on patients' characteristics when a newly diagnosed ONFH patient is confirmed or when an operation is conducted for ONFH patients in each hospital.

Using data from the ONFH sentinel monitoring system over a period of 15 years, a temporal trend of newly diagnosed ONFH patients with respect to basic characteristics were assessed. This included gender ratio, distribution of age at diagnosis, major risk factors, and underlying diseases treated by systemic steroid administration [15]. A total of 3041 newly diagnosed ONFH patients who were reported from 34 collaborating hospitals between 1997 and 2011 were analyzed. The temporal trends of the disease characteristics were assessed in 5-year intervals according to the date of diagnosis (1997–2001, 2002–2006, and 2007–2011). In order to confirm the robustness of the trend, an additional analysis was employed by confining the data to that from 11 hospitals, which regularly reported ONFH patients to the monitoring system throughout the study period.

A notable trend was observed in underlying diseases requiring steroid therapy among ONFH patients with history of systemic steroid use. Across the study period, the proportion of patients with SLE decreased in females (from 1997–2001 to 2007–2011: 37% to 29%, $p = 0.022$). The proportion of patients with renal transplantation also decreased both in males (3.8% to 1.2%, $p = 0.047$) and in females

(3.2% to 0.8%, $p = 0.038$). In contrast, the proportion of patients with pulmonary disease (except for bronchial asthma) increased both in males (0.5% to 5.5%, $p = 0.022$) and in females (0.5% to 3.6%, $p = 0.027$). An increase in the proportion of patients with skin diseases was observed in females (2.2% to 4.4%, $p = 0.046$). Limiting the data to 11 hospitals, additional analysis demonstrated that the results were almost unchanged, although the trends of SLE and renal transplantation were no longer statistically significant due to the reduced number of subjects.

These findings indicate that the distribution of underlying diseases requiring systemic steroid use, which pose a higher risk for ONFH, has gradually changed over time. Current national statistics showed that both the number of SLE patients receiving public financial aid for treatment and the number of patients with renal transplantation have increased in Japan [16, 17]. These trends are inconsistent with those from the ONFH sentinel monitoring system, probably because steroid regimens for SLE treatment or after renal transplantation have evolved so that less are administered [18–20].

A strength of the ONFH monitoring system includes the strict diagnostic criteria because all diagnoses were confirmed by orthopedic hip surgeons who were members of the ONFH Study Group. Less expensive costs and fewer efforts to operate the system in comparison to a nationwide epidemiologic survey are also attractive aspects. For example, as of October 2017, we found that there were 222 newly diagnosed ONFH patients who had been reported to the ONFH sentinel monitoring system, whose diagnosis had been confirmed during 2014. According to the results from the nationwide epidemiologic survey (Table 3.1), the estimated annual number of incident ONFH patients during 2014 in Japan was 2100. Thus, we can expect that newly diagnosed ONFH patients in the ONFH sentinel monitoring system would cover approximately 10% of the incident ONFH patients in Japan overall (222/2100). The ONFH sentinel monitoring system is a useful alternative to evaluate descriptive epidemiology of ONFH both continuously and efficiently.

3.4 Analytic Epidemiology (1): Habitual Alcohol Intake as a Risk Factor

Although descriptive epidemiology of ONFH showed that the history of systemic steroid use and habitual alcohol intake are very prevalent in ONFH patients, analytic epidemiology is required to evaluate whether or not these factors are associated with an increased risk of ONFH.

With respect to evaluation of habitual alcohol intake, a case-control approach is considered particularly suitable because ONFH is a rare disease and a history of alcohol intake in each subject throughout the lifetime can be obtained using a self-administered questionnaire. In Japan, Matsuo et al. were the first to report the association between habitual alcohol intake and ONFH [21]. From 1980 to 1985, they recruited 112 ONFH cases without history of systemic steroid use and 168 matched controls from 4 collaborating hospitals in Japan. They revealed that alcohol drinking status, weekly ethanol consumption, and cumulative ethanol consumption significantly increased the risk of ONFH with evident dose-response relationships. Later, the ONFH Study Group conducted another case-control study where 118 ONFH cases without history of systemic steroid use and 236 matched controls were recruited from 20 collaborating hospitals throughout Japan between 1988 and 1990 [22]. They also found that alcohol drinking status, weekly ethanol consumption, and cumulative ethanol consumption were significantly associated with ONFH. The odds ratios (ORs) were 1.0, 3.2, and 13.1 for former, occasional, and regular drinkers, respectively, in comparison to never drinkers (trend $p < 0.001$); 2.8, 9.4, and 14.8 for <320, 320–799, and ≥800 g/week, respectively, in comparison to nondrinkers (trend $p < 0.001$); 2.2, 9.7, and 12.9 for <3200, 3200–7999, and ≥8000 drink-years, respectively, in comparison to never drinkers (trend $p < 0.001$) (Table 3.3). Similar findings were further confirmed in three case-control studies from Japan [23–25]. The effects of alcohol on ONFH may be immedi-

Table 3.3 Adjusted relative risks of alcohol drinking for ONFH: a case-control study in Japan, 1988–1990

	Cases		Controls			
Characteristics	No.	%	No.	%	Relative odds[a]	95% CI
Alcohol drinking						
Never	23	19.5	87	36.9	1.0	
Former	4	3.4	10	4.2	1.0	0.2–6.2
Occasional	26	22.0	80	33.9	3.2	1.1–9.2
Regular	65	55.1	59	25.0	13.1	4.1–42.5
					Trend: $p < 0.001$	
Weekly ethanol intake (g/week)						
Nondrinker	27	22.9	97	41.1	1.0	
< 320	24	20.3	87	36.9	2.8	1.0–7.8
320–799	49	41.5	45	19.1	9.4	3.0–29.0
≥ 800	18	15.3	7	3.0	14.8	3.8–57.2
					Trend: $p < 0.001$	
Drink-years						
Never drank	23	19.7	87	37.5	1.0	
< 3200	15	12.8	62	26.7	2.2	0.7–6.9
3200–7999	25	21.4	36	15.5	9.7	2.6–36.1
≥ 8000	54	46.2	47	20.3	12.9	3.8–43.4
					Trend: $p < 0.001$	

ONFH idiopathic osteonecrosis of the femoral head, *CI* confidence interval

[a]Adjusted for cigarette smoking, occupational energy consumption, body mass index, and liver dysfunction, using a conditional logistic regression model

ate and cumulative because both current consumption and cumulative consumption increased the risk of ONFH [22].

A recent meta-analysis by Yoon et al. summarized the evidence regarding alcohol intake as a risk factor for ONFH [26]. From 1127 articles which had been published up to January 2016, 5 case-control studies were selected [21–25], all of which were coincidentally Japanese studies and identical to the aforementioned articles. Using the Newcastle-Ottawa Scale (a maximum of 9 stars), the quality assessment showed that each study had a score of 8–9 stars, indicating sufficient quality for evaluation. A conventional meta-analysis to obtain the summary estimate of drinking habits found an increased risk of ONFH among those with former drinkers with marginal significance (OR = 2.62, $p = 0.055$) and a significantly increased risk of ONFH among current drinkers (OR = 3.63, $p < 0.001$ in occasional drinkers; OR = 5.90, $p < 0.001$ in daily drinkers). The dose-response meta-analysis using restricted cubic spline models with four knots revealed that the risk of ONFH significantly increased by 35.3% for every 100 g/week and by 44.1% for every 500 drink-years. Very interestingly, the pattern of dose-response was not J-shaped, but an ever-increasing pattern which indicated that higher alcohol intake resulted in a higher risk of ONFH. In other words, the risk of ONFH is elevated even with a lower alcohol intake level. Since there is no universal consensus regarding the critical dose of alcohol intake which may be necessary for ONFH development, further studies should focus on the threshold of alcohol intake in terms of prevention of ONFH.

3.5 Analytic Epidemiology (2): Systemic Steroid Use as a Risk Factor

To date, associations between systemic steroid use and the risk of ONFH have been assessed mainly among patients with SLE and renal transplantation. However, these findings are not consistent with each other. Information on a complete history of steroid administration in each patient is quite challenging to obtain, especially for total dose and average dose. A single center study may be more convenient for collecting accurate information on steroid therapy compared with a multicenter study, while such a single center study is likely to miss a significant finding due to predefined standard regimens for steroid therapy in each center.

Using a case-control study approach, the ONFH Study Group evaluated systemic steroid use on ONFH risk among SLE patients [4, 27]. They recruited 49 ONFH cases with SLE and 69 matched controls with SLE from 14 collaborating hospitals between 1985 and 1993. Cases and controls were matched for gender, birth year, outpatient department where they received treatment for SLE, and the age at diagnosis of SLE. History of systemic steroid use was collected during the period from the date of diagnosis of SLE to the date of diagnosis of ONFH for cases, and during the period from the date of diagnosis of SLE to the same date of the matched cases for controls. Total dose, maximum dose, and average daily dose were evaluated after being classified into two levels: the lowest and the middle tertile vs. the highest tertile. A significantly elevated OR was found for average daily dose of ≥16.6 mg (vs. < 16.6 mg, OR = 3.7, $p = 0.01$) but not for total dose of ≥28.4 g (vs. < 28.4 g, OR = 2.2, $p = 0.40$) and maximum daily dose of ≥80 mg (vs. < 80 mg, OR = 2.4, $p = 0.06$). With respect to the number of pulse therapies, OR of one dose of pulse therapy was significantly elevated (3.2, $p = 0.02$), while OR of two or more doses of pulse therapy was not significantly associated with ONFH (1.2, $p = 0.80$). Lack of a dose-response relationship between the number of pulse therapies and ONFH risk may indicate that the individual susceptibility to steroids was also associated with ONFH. This interpretation is consistent with a report that patients with lower midazolam clearance showed a significantly higher prevalence of steroid-associated ONFH [28]. Midazolam clearance is a proxy variable of hepatic cytochrome P450 (CYP) 3A, which metabolizes corticosteroids.

The ONFH Study Group also conducted several cohort studies among patients with renal transplantation to evaluate steroid therapy as a risk factor. A study with 150 subjects who received renal transplantation between 1988 and 1999 evaluated the development of ONFH prospectively and routinely using MRI during 1 year after renal transplantation [29]. For total steroid dose during 2 weeks, 4 weeks, 6 weeks and 8 weeks after renal transplantation, a significant association with dose-response relationship was found for total steroid dose during the 8 weeks after renal transplantation (OR of >1795 mg vs. ≤1400 mg: 7.4, $p = 0.01$, trend $p = 0.02$) but not for total steroid dose during 2 weeks, 4 weeks, and 6 weeks. In contrast, the same study with 286 subjects in which recruitment period had been extended until 2007 showed that the most pronounced association with dose-response relationship was found for total steroid dose during the 2 week period after renal transplantation (OR of >600 mg vs. ≤520 mg: 4.9, $p < 0.01$, trend $p < 0.01$) [30].

Although patients with SLE or renal transplantation seem to be suitable populations for evaluating systemic steroid use on ONFH risk, they can only provide effect estimates comparing high doses and low doses of steroids. Thus, the ONFH Study Group conducted another case-control study to evaluate the extent of ONFH risk between steroid users and non-steroid users. They recruited 73 ONFH cases irrespective of history of systemic steroid use and 250 matched controls and found that history of oral corticosteroid use was significantly associated with development of ONFH approximately 20-fold [31]. Using a very similar dataset, interactions between oral corticosteroid use and alcohol intake were evaluated [25]. Among 71 ONFH cases and 227 matched controls, multiplicative interaction and additive interaction were assessed using a two-by-two table of "nondrinker vs. drinker" for alcohol intake and "never-user vs. user" for oral corticosteroids. When nondrinkers without steroid use were set as a reference group, an elevated but non-significant OR was observed for drinkers without steroid use (OR: 2.79). In contrast, nondrinkers with steroid use showed a substantially elevated OR (OR: 31.5). However, no further increase in OR was observed for drinkers with steroid use (OR: 31.6). Consequently, any significant multiplicative or additive interaction was

Table 3.4 Multiplicative or additive interaction between current drinking status and history of oral corticosteroid use for ONFH: a case-control study in Japan, 2002–2004

	Never user of oral corticosteroids		User of oral corticosteroids			
Variables	Cases (n)/controls (n)	Adjusted OR (95% CI)[c]	Cases (n)/controls (n)	Adjusted OR (95% CI)[c]	*p*-value for multiplicative interaction[a]	Synergy index[b] (95% CI)
Current drinking status						
Nondrinker	4/79	1	22/15	31.5 (9.05–109)		
Drinker	23/122	2.79 (0.89–8.77)	22/11	31.6 (8.67–115)	0.19	0.95 (0.32–2.80)

ONFH idiopathic osteonecrosis of the femoral head, *OR* odds ratio, *CI* confidence interval

[a]Wald test for each interaction term (DF = 1)

[b]Synergy index >1 indicates additive interaction

[c]Adjusted for gender, age, smoking and past history of liver disease, hyperlipidemia and gout, using a logistic regression model

detected (Table 3.4). Although pharmacokinetic interactions between steroids and alcohol is possible, the most plausible interpretation may be that the added effect of alcohol intake was too small to make any significant difference in the presence of the overwhelming effect of steroids on ONFH risk. Together with the findings from descriptive epidemiology in which ONFH is frequently observed among middle-aged individuals and younger ONFH cases are likely to have a greater history of systemic steroid use, the development of preventative strategies especially for steroid-associated ONFH is urgently sought.

3.6 Summary

The ONFH Study Group and the ERID Study Groups have conducted a variety of epidemiologic studies together and have systematically elucidated the epidemiology of ONFH in Japan. Although the underlying mechanisms of ONFH are still controversial, epidemiologic findings can contribute to policy and provide a clue for experimental or clinical studies regarding pathogenesis and effective treatment. Several methodologies that have been proposed by the ERID research group could be helpful in understanding epidemiology on other intractable diseases. Regarding ONFH, specific issues to be evaluated in further epidemiologic studies include periodic updating of descriptive epidemiology, determining "safe" thresholds of alcohol intake and steroid dosages for elevated risk of ONFH, while other potential factors associated with ONFH should also be explored. Continuous efforts to collaborate effectively between the ONFH Study Group and the ERID Study Groups should result in accumulation of further evidence.

References

1. Lavernia CJ, Sierra RJ, Grieco FR. Osteonecrosis of the femoral head. J Am Acad Orthop Surg. 1999;7:250–61.
2. Assouline-Dayan Y, Chang C, Greenspan A, Shoenfeld Y, Gershwin ME. Pathogenesis and natural history of osteonecrosis. Semin Arthritis Rheum. 2002;32:94–124.
3. Mont MA, Cherian JJ, Sierra RJ, Jones LC, Lieberman JR. Nontraumatic osteonecrosis of the femoral head: where do we stand today? A ten-year update. J Bone Joint Surg Am. 2015;97:1604–27.
4. Hirota Y, Hotokebuchi T, Sugioka Y. Idiopathic osteonecrosis of the femoral head: nationwide epidemiologic studies in Japan. In: Urbaniak JR, Jones Jr JP, editors. Osteonecrosis -- etiology, diagnosis and treatment. Rosemont: American Academy of Orthopaedic surgeons; 1997. p. 51–8.
5. Yanagawa H. [Recent progress of epidemiological studies on intractable diseases in Japan] [in Japanese]. Nihon Eiseigaku Zasshi. 1995;49:950–9.
6. Hashimoto S, Fukutomi K, Nagai M, Nakamura Y, Yanagawa H, Sasaki R, Ohno Y. [A note on methods for estimating the number of patients in the nationwide epidemiological survey on intractable diseases] [in Japanese]. Nihon Koshu Eisei Zasshi. 1990;37:768–74.
7. Hashimoto S, Fukutomi K, Nagai M, Nakamura Y, Yanagawa H, Sasaki R, Ohno Y, Kubo N, Aoki K. [A method of interval estimation for number of patients in the nationwide epidemiological survey on intractable diseases] [in Japanese]. Nihon Koshu Eisei Zasshi. 1991;38:880–3.
8. Nakamura Y, Matsumoto T, Tamakoshi A, Kawamura T, Seino Y, Kasuga M, Yanagawa H, Ohno Y. Prevalence of idiopathic hypoparathyroidism and pseudohypoparathyroidism in Japan. J Epidemiol. 2000;10:29–33.
9. Nakamura Y. [A manual of a nationwide epidemiologic survey for estimating the number of patients and assessing clinico-epidemiological characteristics of patients with intractable diseases (3rd edition)] [in Japanese]. The Study Group on Epidemiologic Research for Intractable Diseases. 2017. http://www.jichi.ac.jp/dph/nanbyou/manual_2017.pdf. Accessed 31 Oct 2017.
10. Aoki R, Ohno Y, Tamakoshi A, Kawamura T, Wakai K, Senda M, Lin YS, Ninomiya S, Hirota Y, Igarashi Y, Hashimoto S, Aizawa S, Minowa M, Inaba Y. [Nationwide epidemiological survey on idiopathic osteonecrosis of the femoral head in Japan] [in Japanese]. Tokyo: The Annual Report of the Study Group on Epidemiologic Research for Intractable Diseases in the fiscal year of 1995, Ministry of Health of Japan.; 1996. p. 67–72.
11. Fukushima W, Fujioka M, Kubo T, Tamakoshi A, Nagai M, Hirota Y. Nationwide epidemiologic survey of idiopathic osteonecrosis of the femoral head. Clin Orthop Relat Res. 2010;468:2715–24.
12. Fukushima W, Sakai T, Nakamura Y, Sugano N. [Nationwide epidemiologic survey on idiopathic osteonecrosis of the femoral head in Japan] [in Japanese]. Tokyo: The Annual Report of the Study Group on Idiopathic Osteonecrosis of the Femoral Head in the fiscal year of 2016, Ministry of Health and Welfare of Japan. 2017. http://mhlw-grants.niph.go.jp/niph/search/NIDD00.do?resrchNum=201610024B. Accessed 31 Oct 2017.
13. Sugano N, Atsumi T, Ohzono K, Kubo T, Hotokebuchi T, Takaoka K. The 2001 revised criteria for diagnosis, classification, and staging of idiopathic osteonecrosis of the femoral head. J Orthop Sci. 2002;7:601–5.

14. Sugano N, Kubo T, Takaoka K, Ohzono K, Hotokebuchi T, Matsumoto T, Igarashi H, Ninomiya S. Diagnostic criteria for non-traumatic osteonecrosis of the femoral head. A multicentre study. J Bone Joint Surg Br. 1999;81:590–5.
15. Takahashi S, Fukushima W, Yamamoto T, Iwamoto Y, Kubo T, Sugano N, Hirota Y. Japanese sentinel monitoring study Group for Idiopathic Osteonecrosis of the femoral head. Temporal trends in characteristics of newly diagnosed nontraumatic osteonecrosis of the femoral head from 1997 to 2011: a hospital-based sentinel monitoring system in Japan. J Epidemiol. 2015;25:437–44.
16. Japan Intractable Diseases Information Center: The number of cases of intractable diseases in Japan [in Japanese]. http://www.nanbyou.or.jp/entry/1356. Accessed 31 Oct 2017.
17. Japan Organ Transplant Network: Donors and Transplants Data. http://www.jotnw.or.jp/english/data.html. Accessed 31 Oct 2017.
18. Houssiau FA, Ginzler EM. Current treatment of lupus nephritis. Lupus. 2008;17:426–30.
19. Kumar MS, Heifets M, Moritz MJ, Saeed MI, Khan SM, Fyfe B, Sustento-Riodeca N, Daniel JN, Kumar A. Safety and efficacy of steroid withdrawal two days after kidney transplantation: analysis of results at three years. Transplantation. 2006;81:832–9.
20. Arnol M, de Mattos AM, Chung JS, Prather JC, Mittalhenkle A, Norman DJ. Late steroid withdrawal and cardiovascular events in kidney transplant recipients. Transplantation. 2008;86:1844–8.
21. Matsuo K, Hirohata T, Sugioka Y, Ikeda M, Fukuda A. Influence of alcohol intake, cigarette smoking, and occupational status on idiopathic osteonecrosis of the femoral head. Clin Orthop Relat Res. 1988;234:115–23.
22. Hirota Y, Hirohata T, Fukuda K, Mori M, Yanagawa H, Ohno Y, Sugioka Y. Association of alcohol intake, cigarette smoking, and occupational status with the risk of idiopathic osteonecrosis of the femoral head. Am J Epidemiol. 1993;137:530–8.
23. Shibata A, Fukuda K, Inoue A, Higuchi F, Miyake H, Nishi M, Mori M, Ishii S, Nagao M, Yanagawa H. Flushing pattern and idiopathic avascular necrosis of the femoral head. J Epidemiol. 1996;6:37–43.
24. Sakata R. A case-control study of association between life-style, alcohol dehydrogenase 2 and aldehyde dehydrogenase 2 genotype and idiopathic osteonecrosis of the femoral head. Kurume Med J. 2003;50:121–30.
25. Fukushima W, Yamamoto T, Takahashi S, Sakaguchi M, Kubo T, Iwamoto Y, Hirota Y. The effect of alcohol intake and the use of oral corticosteroids on the risk of idiopathic osteonecrosis of the femoral head: a case-control study in Japan. Bone Joint J. 2013;95-B:320–5.
26. Yoon BH, Kim TY, Shin IS, Lee HY, Lee YJ, Koo KH. Alcohol intake and the risk of osteonecrosis of the femoral head in Japanese populations: a dose-response meta-analysis of case-control studies. Clin Rheumatol. 2017;36:2517–24.
27. Ohzono K, Lee K, Ando W, Takao M, Sugano N, Nishii T, Hirota Y. Predictors for corticosteroid associated osteonecrosis of the femoral head among patients with sustemic lupus erythematosus [in Japanese]. Riumachika. 2002;27:114–7.
28. Kaneshiro Y, Oda Y, Iwakiri K, Masada T, Iwaki H, Hirota Y, Kondo K, Takaoka K. Low hepatic cytochrome P450 3A activity is a risk for corticosteroid-induced osteonecrosis. Clin Pharmacol Ther. 2006;80:396–402.
29. Shibatani M, Fujioka M, Arai Y, Takahashi K, Ueshima K, Okamoto M, Yoshimura N, Hirota Y, Fukushima W, Kubo T. Degree of corticosteroid treatment within the first 2 months of renal transplantation has a strong influence on the incidence of osteonecrosis of the femoral head. Acta Orthop. 2008;79:631–6.
30. Saito M, Ueshima K, Fujioka M, Ishida M, Goto T, Arai Y, Ikoma K, Fujiwara H, Fukushima W, Kubo T. Corticosteroid administration within 2 weeks after renal transplantation affects the incidence of femoral head osteonecrosis. Acta Orthop. 2014;85:266–70.
31. Sakaguchi M, Tanaka T, Fukushima W, Kubo T, Hirota Y. Idiopathic ONF Multicenter Case-Control Study Group. Impact of oral corticosteroid use for idiopathic osteonecrosis of the femoral head: a nationwide multicenter case-control study in Japan. J Orthop Sci. 2010;15:185–91.

Chapter 4
Risk Factors in Amyotrophic Lateral Sclerosis

Kazushi Okamoto

Abstract Amyotrophic lateral sclerosis (ALS) is a devastating and lethal adult-onset degenerative disease of the upper and lower motor neuron systems. It is of unknown etiology and affects the motor neurons in the spinal cord, leading to atrophy of the skeletal muscles, paralysis, and death within 2–5 years of symptom onset, often due to respiratory insufficiency. High incidence areas are located approximately on the 135 east longitude. Most cases of ALS are sporadic, with only 5–10% having a family history, suggesting that nongenetic factors have a greater effect on the development of ALS than genetic factors.

In this review, we introduce the major factors related to the development of ALS and provide data on gender and age group differences for the risk factors listed.

Keywords Amyotrophic lateral sclerosis · Risk factors · Lifestyle · Environment Medical condition

4.1 Introduction

Amyotrophic lateral sclerosis (ALS) is a progressive neurodegenerative disease of unclear etiology, which involves the motor neurons of the spinal cord, rapidly progressing to atrophy of skeletal muscles, paralysis, and death.

Although familial ALS can be inherited in an autosomal dominant, autosomal recessive, or X-linked manner [1, 2], sporadic ALS accounts for over 90%

K. Okamoto
Department of Public Health and Epidemiology, Aichi Prefectural College School of Nursing and Health, Nagoya, Japan
e-mail: okamoto@nrs.aichi-pu.ac.jp

M. Washio, G. Kobashi (eds.), *Epidemiological Studies of Specified Rare and Intractable Disease*, Current Topics in Environmental Health and Preventive Medicine, https://doi.org/10.1007/978-981-13-1096-6_4

of the cases [3], suggesting complex environmental and genetic factors are involved. The disease is classified in two categories based on the manner of onset: limb onset (80% cases) or bulbar onset (20% cases). In the former, symptoms appear distally or proximally in the upper or lower limb, while the latter usually manifests with dysarthria and dysphagia, with limb symptoms presenting at the same time or later in the course of the disease [4]. About 50% of patients with ALS die within 30 months of symptom onset, often from respiratory insufficiency [2].

The incidence of sporadic ALS shows little variation in the world, ranging from 1 to 2 per 100,000 person-years [5, 6]. According to Marin et al. [7], the overall pooled crude incidence of ALS worldwide is 1.75 (1.55–1.96) per 100,000 person-years, being more prevalent in men (2.03 (1.79–2.37) vs. 1.45 (1.25–1.64) in women) with a male-to-female ratio of 1.2–1.5 [7, 8]. The rates range from 2.35 (1.79–2.92) in West Europe to a low 0.78 (0.5–1.05) in East Asia [7]. The pooled incidence from European subcontinents ranged from 1.92 (1.49–2.34) in North Europe (number of studies, $n = 11$), to 2.22 (1.72–2.73) in South Europe ($n = 9$), and 2.35 (1.79–2.92) in West Europe ($n = 4$), per 100,000 person-years, while the incidence was at 1.59 (1.32–1.87) for North America ($n = 10$) and 0.78 (0.50–1.05) for East Asia ($n = 3$) [7]. It is worth mentioning that the prevalence of ALS is 50–100 times higher in the geographical area located at approximately 135 degrees east longitude, namely in Guam, Papua-New Guinea, and Kii peninsula of Honshu island in Japan [9–11]. The crude average annual incidence in Wakayama prefecture, in the Kii peninsula, is 2.50/100000 (male 3.08, female 1.99). Even so, ALS prevalence is much higher than average in Kozagawa and Koza areas (10.56 (male 14.14, female 7.66) per 100,000) [9]. This is much lower than the rate reported in these areas by the end of 2002, with an overall prevalence of 11.31 (male 14.40, female 8.53) in Wakayama prefecture and 52.81 (male 70.70, female 38.28) in Kozagawa and Koza areas [9]. ALS is rarely observed before the age of 40, and the incidence increases with age thereafter, with the mean age at onset being 58–63 years for sporadic ALS and 40–60 years for familial ALS [12, 13].

4.2 General Overview of Risk Factors for ALS

4.2.1 Familial Tendency

Early case-control studies found that families with ALS patients had threefold [14] to over tenfold risk [15] of ALS. Pooling several twin registers from Sweden and the UK, the heritability for ALS is estimated to be 61% [16].

4.2.2 *Genetic Factors*

4.2.2.1 SOD1

Although ALS is predominantly a sporadic disease, 10% of cases are described as familial (fALS). Historically, SOD1 (Copper-Zinc-superoxide dismutase) is known to play a role in the classic adult-onset fALS. The most common SOD1 mutation worldwide is inherited in both dominant and recessive manners [17, 18].

4.2.2.2 Chromosome 9

A mutation in this Chromosome 9 has been shown to segregate with both ALS and frontal temporal dementia in studies of American, European, and Japanese patients [19–22]. Recently, the repeat expansion of Chromosome 9 was higher in ALS patients in the Kii Peninsula of Japan (20%) than the rest of Japan (less than 2.5%), indicating that it may partially account for the incidence of ALS-PDC in this geographic focus [22].

4.2.3 *Lifestyle Factors*

4.2.3.1 Body Mass Index (BMI)

ALS patients have a lower BMI and less intake of total energy and protein than controls [23] and this has been shown to be an independent prognostic indicator for ALS after diagnosis. Longitudinal cohort studies suggest that premorbid underweight male subjects were at a significantly higher risk of ALS compared to normal-weight men [24].

4.2.3.2 Smoking

There is no clear association between smoking and ALS. Alonso et al. reported a pooled relative risk (RR) (95% confidence interval (CI)) of 1.28 (0.97–1.68) for current smokers compared to never smokers and 1.12 (0.98–1.27) for former versus never and former smokers for ALS [25], with an estimated RR (95% CI] of 0.86 (0.71–1.03) in men and 1.66 (1.31–2.10) in women [25]. On the other hand, Okamoto et al. [23], Kamel et al. [15], and Pamphlett et al. [26] reported no significant association between smoking and ALS. In another study, smoking was believed to result in a lower survival rate in women but not in men [27].

4.2.3.3 Alcohol Consumption

Alonso et al. [25] estimated the odds ratio (OR) for the association between alcohol consumption and ALS to be 0.57 (95% CI; 0.51–0.64), suggesting that alcohol consumption reduced the risk for developing ALS, while there was no significant relationship [24].

4.2.3.4 Head Injury

Peters et al. reported a moderately elevated risk of ALS among individuals with previous head injuries (OR = 1.7, 95 percent CI; 1.3, 2.2) [28]. Binazzi et al. also suggested an association between severe head injury of less than 1 year before diagnosis of ALS (OR: 3.9, 95% CI 2.6–6.1) [29]. Although they suggested older injuries (11–30 years prior) might be associated with bulbar onset ALS [29]. In another study, no significant increase in ALS was observed in people with head injuries more than 3 years prior to the onset of symptoms [30]. In a large population-based study, Pupillo et al. [31] reported that repeated traumatic events occurring at least 5 years before diagnosis were associated with an increased rate of ALS (OR 2.6 for three or more events). Chio et al. also confirmed that bulbar onset type of the disease is more common among Italian soccer players with ALS [32]. Trauma-related neuro-inflammation and microglial activation, disruption of the blood brain barrier, mitochondrial dysfunction and excessive oxidative and nitric radicals, and the accumulation of tau protein are suggested to be mechanisms inducing ALS following head injuries [33, 34].

4.2.3.5 Physical Activity

No definite relationship has been described between physical activity and risk of ALS [35].

Although one study suggests that a highly active lifestyle and vigorous activity lead to at an increased risk for ALS [36].

According to Longstreth WT et al. [37], vigorous physical activity could potentiate the effect of a toxin to motor neurons through several mechanisms, especially if the toxin's effects were mediated through nerve cell excitation. Previous findings also point to an increased risk of ALS professional football players [38, 39], but not in high school players [40]. Even so, a large European case-control study showed that physical activity (adjustment OR = 0.65, 95% CI = 0.48–0.89), whether work-related (adjustment OR = 0.56, 95% CI = 0.36–0.87) or organized sports (adjustment OR = 0.49, 95% CI = 0.32–0.75), was associated with reduced odds of developing ALS [41]. Ingre C et al. suggest that different levels of physical exercise (professional vs. recreational) may have very different biological effect on neurodegeneration [42].

4.2.4 Oxidative Status

4.2.4.1 Type A Personality

Type A personality refers to an individual who is impatient, excessively time-conscious, status insecure, highly competitive, hostile, aggressive, and incapable of relaxation. They are often highly achieving workaholics who multitask, drive themselves with deadlines, and are unhappy about the smallest of delays. Dissatisfaction and stress are related to more frequent complaints in Type A individuals [43]. There is a significantly higher relation between role conflict and physical and psychological strain in those with Type A personalities than those with Type B [44].

Okamoto K et al. reported that a Type A behavioral pattern was not only associated with a significant overall increased ALS risk but also in all gender and age group combinations (<65 year vs. ≥65 years) [45], which could be due to increased endogenous oxidative stress for the nervous system in these individuals.

The combination of a type A behavior pattern and low intake of green-yellow vegetables is suggested to have the greatest effect on the risk for ALS (adjusted OR, 11.2; 95% CI, 3.8–33.0), pointing to a role for oxidants in ALS either in the form of patient-specific factors and/or diminished or missing antioxidant defense system in motor neurons [23].

4.2.4.2 8-Hydroxydeoxyguanosine (8-OHdG)

8-Hydroxydeoxyguanosine (8-OHdG) is produced by the reaction of reactive oxygen species (ROS) and guanine residues in the DNA, which if not reverted by intracellular antioxidant agents, is excised and secreted in the plasma, from where it will be excreted in the urine [46, 47]. Hence, in recent years urinary level of 8-OHdG is considered a biomarker for oxidative damage to the DNA [48, 49].

Urinary 8-OHdG excretion increases with age and H-Y staging of the patients with Parkinson disease, and reflects increased systemic levels of oxidative DNA damage that is caused by mitochondrial dysfunction in skeletal muscles [48].

8-OHdG levels were higher in Kii than in other areas in Japan [50]. The mean level of 8-OHdG in Oshima residents, who changed the source of their drinking water to the Kozagawa River in 1975, was higher than that of controls ($p < 0.05$) [50]. Besides, the morning spot urinary 8-OHdG and 8-OHdG/creatinine levels were significantly higher in the patients with ALS in the K area than in controls [50]. The mean urinary 8-OHdG/creatinine ratio of Kii patients with ALS/PD was higher than that of age-matched control subjects [51].

4.2.5 *Metals*

4.2.5.1 Calcium (Ca) and Magnesium (Mg)

Traditionally, it was believed that low concentration of calcium and magnesium in drinking and river water was associated with high incidence of motor neuron disease (MND) in the area [52, 53].

K-area, which has a high incidence of ALS, has markedly low levels of Ca and Mg in the drinking water [54]. Residents in K area also have lower serum Ca than control subjects from other areas [54].

4.2.5.2 Copper (Zn) and Zinc (Cu)

Low serum Zn and Cu levels, high Cu/Zn ratios, and high urinary 8-OHdG levels were commonly found in the patients with ALS in the Kii area and the Oshima residents [54].

Serum Zn levels were negatively correlated with serum Cu levels in the patients with ALS, while the serum Cu levels exhibited a tendency towards a positive correlation with urinary 8-OHdG/creatinine level [54]. Kihira et al. found that patients with ALS in the K area (K-ALS) and non-patient residents (K residents) had lower serum Cu and Zn levels and Cu/Zn ratio compared to control subjects from other areas [54].

In experimental studies, Zn deficiency has been reported to affect DNA damage and DNA repair [55], weaken the antioxidant defense system, and increase oxidative stress in rat erythrocytes [56]. Significant increased levels of Cu ion have been found in the spinal cord of an ALS mouse model.

4.2.5.3 Manganese (Mn) and Aluminum (Al)

Yase reported on the correlation between high concentration of manganese (Mn) and high incidence of MND in Kozagawa and Guam. Epidemiological studies have shown that garden soil contained high amounts of Al and Mn in redsidents in K area [52, 53]. Mg and vanadium levels were also higher in the scalp hair of patients with K-ALS than those of control subjects [50].

Mn is well known to have neurotoxic properties [56], and Mn concentrations in CSF samples of ALS patients were significantly elevated compared to healthy controls [57].

4.2.5.4 Environmental Change

In Oshima, no patients had been reported with ALS between 1960 and 1999. The recent increase in the number of ALS patients in this region is attributed to resourcing the drinking water for that region from the Kozagawa River since 1975

[55]. In this population the level of Ca, Mg, Cu, and Zn is significantly lower, while the oxidative stress markers (8-OHdG) is close to the level observed in the mainland K area, suggesting a role for such an environmental change in the development of ALS [54].

4.3 Nutritional Status

4.3.1 Macronutrients

A high intake of carbohydrate was associated with an increased risk of ALS, while that of total fat, saturated fatty acids (SFAs), monounsaturated fatty acids (MUFAs), and polyunsaturated fatty acids (PUFAs) reduced the risk of ALS significantly [58].

This might be due to the production of free radicals, oxidant stress, and reactive oxygen species leading to apoptotic cell death due to high glucose levels [59], while a diet high in fat seems to have a neuroprotective effect [60, 61].

4.3.2 Dietary Intake of Antioxidant Rich Food

Russo et al., and Luyer et al., demonstrated that the increase of intake of fruit and vegetables may protect against oxidative stress by strengthening the radical scavenger system [62]. A high intake of the five antioxidant-rich food groups (green-yellow vegetables, fruits, mushroom, seaweed, and dairy products), especially green-yellow vegetables, was associated with a significant decrease in the risk of ALS (≥2 vs. none adjusted OR: 0.33 95% CI; 0.18–0.60) by about 70% [63] (Table 4.1). Higher antioxidant intake score as index of intake frequency and number of food group with antioxidant-rich food consumed was associated with a reduced risk of ALS [64].

Table 4.1 Adjusted OR[a] and 95% CI for ALS according to antioxidant intake score [63]

Dietary antioxidants score	Cases ($n = 143$)	Controls ($n = 385$)	Crude odds ratio	95% CI	Adjusted[a] odds ratio	95% CI
Lowest	32.9%	20.5%	1.00	(reference)	1.00	(reference)
Medium	38.5	35.3	0.90	0.59–1.37	0.84	0.54–1.33
Highest	28.7	44.2	0.30	0.16–0.54	0.31	0.17–0.57
P for trend			$p = 0.0001$		$p = 0.0001$	

[a]Adjusted for sex, age, Type A behavior pattern

4.3.3 *Antioxidant Vitamins*

4.3.3.1 Vitamin E

Vitamin E intake is associated with reduced risk of ALS, but there was no statistically significant association reported in case-control study [63] and in 5 Prospective Cohort Studies [65].

4.3.3.2 Other Vitamins

Okamoto et al. reported that a higher intake of β-carotene significantly reduced the risk of ALS (lowest vs. highest; OR = 0.66; 95% CI 0.35–1.23) [63].

4.3.3.3 Dietary Patterns

A healthy dietary pattern characterized by high loadings for green and yellow vegetables, seaweed, pulses, other vegetables, mushrooms, dairy products, fruits, fish, soy products, and Japanese and Chinese tea was associated with a significantly reduced risk for ALS, revealing that those in the highest percentile of Healthy pattern showed reduction of about 65% in risk for ALS [66].

4.4 Differences in Risk Factors Based on Gender and Age Group

Okamoto et al. reported that Type A behavior pattern was significantly associated with an increased risk for ALS in all gender and age group combinations (<65 year vs. ≥65 years), indicating that Type A behavior, as a patient-specific endogenous oxidative stress, may enhance the common ALS risks in all gender and age group combinations. Less frequent intake of green vegetables in men 65 years and over, vigorous exercise in men younger than 65 years, and self-reported stress in both men and women aged ≥65 years were associated with an increased ALS risk.

Summary of differences in risk factors by gender and age groups is shown in Tables 4.2 and 4.3.

Table 4.2 Differences in risk factors by gender and age groups [45]

	Males		Females	
	<65 years	≥65 years	<65 years	≥65 years
Chronic physical stress (vigorous exercise)	+			
Stress-producing behavior (type A behavior pattern)	+	+	+	+
Acute psychological stress (much self-reported stress)		+		+
Less anti-oxidative protective system (less intake of green-yellow vegetable)	+	±	+	+

+: convince factor ±: possible factor

Table 4.3 Risk factors and preventive factors for the development of amyotrophic lateral sclerosis (ALS)

Risk factors	Association with the development of ALS	References
Lifestyles		
Low BMI	Positive	[23, 24]
Current smoker	No association	[15, 25–27]
Current drinker	No association/inverse	[24, 25]
Head injury	No association/positive	[28–34]
Physical activity	Inverse	[35–42]
Oxidative stress		
Type A behavior pattern personality	Positive	[23, 43–45]
8-OHdG	Positive	[46–51]
Concentration of metals in blood		
Low calcium	Positive	[52–54]
Low magnesium	Positive	
Low zinc	Positive	[54–56]
Low cupper	Positive	
High manganese	Positive	[50, 52, 53, 56, 57]
High aluminum	Positive	
Dietary factors		
Carbohydrate	Positive	[58–61]
Fats, fatty acids	Inverse	
SFA, MUFA, PUFA	Inverse	
Protein	Inverse	
Antioxidants rich in food intake		
Fruits	Inverse	[63]
Green/yellow vegs	Inverse	
Antioxidants intake score	Inverse	[64]
Antioxidant vitamin intake		
β-Carotene	Inverse	[63]
Vitamin C	No association	[63]
Vitamin E	No association/	[63, 65]
Dietary pattern		
Healthy pattern	Inverse	[66]
Traditional pattern	Positive	

References

1. Maruyama H, Morino H, Ito H, Izumi Y, Kato H, Watanabe Y, et al. Mutations of optineurin in amyotrophic lateral sclerosis. Nature. 2010;465:223–6.
2. Turner MR, Hardiman O, Benatar M, Brooks BR, Chio A, de Carvalho M, et al. Controversies and priorities in amyotrophic lateral sclerosis. Lancet Neurol. 2013;12:310–22.
3. Gellera C, Castellotti B, Riggio MC, Silani V, Morandi L, Testa D, et al. Superoxide dismutase gene mutations in Italian patients with familial and sporadic amyotrophic lateral sclerosis: identification of three novel missense mutations. Neuromuscul Disord. 2001;11:404–10.
4. Appel SH, Zhao W, Beers DR, Henkel JS. The microglial-motoneuron dialogue in ALS. Acta Myol. 2011;30:4–8.
5. McGuire V, Longstreth WT Jr, Koepsell TD, van Belle G. Incidence of amyotrophic lateral sclerosis in three counties in western Washington state. Neurology. 1996;47(2):571–3.
6. Traynor BJ, Codd MB, Corr B, Forde C, Frost E, Hardiman O. Incidence and prevalence of ALS in Ireland, 1995–1997: a population-based study. Neurology. 1999;52(3):504–9.
7. Marin B, Boumédiene F, Logroscino G, Couratier P, Babron MC, Leutenegger AL, et al. Variation in worldwide incidence of amyotrophic lateral sclerosis: a meta-analysis. Int J Epidemiol. 2017 Feb 1;46(1):57–74.
8. Manjaly ZR, Scott KM, Abhinav K, et al. The sex ratio in amyotrophic lateral sclerosis: a population based study. Amyotroph Lateral Scler. 2010;11(5):439–42.
9. Kihira T, Yoshida S, Hironishi M, Miwa H, Okamato K, Kondo T. Changes in the incidence of amyotrophic lateral sclerosis in Wakayama, Japan. Amyotroph Lateral Scler Other Motor Neuron Disord. 2005 Sep;6(3):155–63.
10. Sejvar JJ, Holman RC, Bresee JS, Kochanek KD, Schonberger LB. Amyotrophic lateral sclerosis mortality in the United States, 1979–2001. Neuroepidemiology. 2005;25(3):144–52.
11. Plato CC, Garruto RM, Galasko D, et al. Amyotrophic lateral sclerosis and parkinsonism-dementia complex of Guam: changing incidence rates during the past 60 years. Am J Epidemiol. 2003;157(2):149–57.
12. Testa D, Lovati R, Ferrarini M, Salmoiraghi F, Filippini G. Survival of 793 patients with amyotrophic lateral sclerosis diagnosed over a 28-year period. Amyotroph Lateral Scler Other Motor Neuron Disord. 2004;5(4):208–12.
13. Logroscino G, Traynor BJ, Hardiman O, et al. Incidence of amyotrophic lateral sclerosis in Europe. J Neurol Neurosurg Psychiatry. 2010;81(4):385–90.
14. Cruz DC, Nelson LM, McGuire V, Longstreth WT Jr. Physical trauma and family history of neurodegenerative diseases in amyotrophic lateral sclerosis: a population-based case-control study. Neuroepidemiology. 1999;18(2):101–10.
15. Kamel F, Umbach DM, Munsat TL, Shefner JM, Sandler DP. Association of cigarette smoking with amyotrophic lateral sclerosis. Neuroepidemiology. 1999;18(4):194–202.
16. Al-Chalabi A, Fang F, Hanby MF, Leigh PN, Shaw CE, Ye W, et al. An estimate of amyotrophic lateral sclerosis heritability using twin data. J Neurol Neurosurg Psychiatry. 2010;81(12):1324–6.
17. Robberecht W, Aguirre T, Van den Bosch L, Tilkin P, Cassiman JJ, Matthijs G. D90A heterozygosity in the SOD1 gene is associated with familial and apparently sporadic amyotrophic lateral sclerosis. Neurology. 1996;47(5):1336–9.
18. Andersen P. Amyotrophic lateral sclerosis associated with mutations in the CuZn superoxide dismutase gene. Curr Neurol Neurosci Rep. 2006;6(1):37–46.
19. Renton AE, Majounie E, Waite A, et al. A hexanucleotide repeat expansion in C9ORF72 is the cause of chromosome 9p21-linked ALS-FTD. Neuron. 2011;72(2):257–68.
20. Gijselinck I, Van Langenhove T, van der Zee J, et al. A C9orf72 promoter repeat expansion in a Flanders-Belgian cohort with disorders of the frontotemporal lobar degeneration-amyotrophic lateral sclerosis spectrum: a gene identification study. Lancet Neurol. 2012;11(1):54–65.

21. Millecamps S, Boillée S, Le Ber I, et al. Phenotype difference between ALS patients with expanded repeats in C9ORF72 and patients with mutations in other ALS-related genes. J Med Genet. 2012;49(4):258–63.
22. Ishiura H, Takahashi Y, Mitsui J, Yoshida S, Kihira T, Kokubo Y, et al. C9ORF72 repeat expansion in amyotrophic lateral sclerosis in the Kii peninsula of Japan. Arch Neurol. 2012;69(9):1154–8.
23. Okamoto K, Kihira T, Kondo T, Kobashi G, Washio M, Sasaki S, et al. Lifestyle factors and risk of amyotrophic lateral sclerosis: a case-control study in Japan. Ann Epidemiol. 2009;19(6):359–64. https://doi.org/10.1016/j.annepidem.2009.01.015. Epub 2009 Apr 2
24. Gallo V, Wark PA, Jenab M, Pearce N, Brayne C, Vermeulen R, et al. Prediagnostic body fat and risk of death from amyotrophic lateral sclerosis: the EPIC cohort. Neurology. 2013 Feb 26;80(9):829–38. https://doi.org/10.1212/WNL.0b013e3182840689.
25. Alonso A, Logroscino G, Hernán MA. Smoking and the risk of amyotrophic lateral sclerosis: a systematic review and meta-analysis. J Neurol Neurosurg Psychiatry. 2010;81(11):1249–52.
26. Pamphlett R, Ward EC. Smoking is not a risk factor for sporadic amyotrophic lateral sclerosis in an Australian population. Neuroepidemiology. 2012;38(2):106–13.
27. Alonso A, Logroscino G, Jick SS, Hernán MA. Association of smoking with amyotrophic lateral sclerosis risk and survival in men and women: a prospective study. BMC Neurol. 2010 Jan 14;10:6.
28. Peters ME, Rao V, Bechtold KT, Roy D, Sair HI, Leoutsakos JM, et al. Head injury serum markers for assessing response to trauma: design of the HeadSMART study. Brain Inj. 2017;31(3):370–8.
29. Binazzi A, Belli S, Uccelli R, Desiato MT, Talamanca IF, Antonini G, et al. An exploratory case control study on spinal and bulbar forms of amyotrophic lateral sclerosis in the province of Rome. Amyotroph Lateral Scler. 2009 Oct-Dec;10(5–6):361–9.
30. Peters TL, Fang F, Weibull CE, Sandler DP, Kamel F, Ye W. Severe head injury and amyotrophic lateral sclerosis. Amyotroph Lateral Scler Frontotemporal Degener. 2013;14(4):267–72.
31. Beghi E, Logroscino G, Micheli A, Millul A, Perini M, Riva R, et al. Validity of hospital discharge diagnoses for the assessment of the prevalence and incidence of amyotrophic lateral sclerosis. Amyotrophic Lateral Scler. 2001;2:99–104.
32. Chen H, Richard M, Sandler DP, Umbach DM, Kamel F. Head injury and amyotrophic lateral sclerosis. Am J Epidemiol. 2007;166(7):810–6.
33. Szczygielski J, Mautes A, Steudel WI, Falkai P, Bayer TA, Wirths O. Traumatic brain injury: cause or risk of Alzheimer's disease? A review of experimental studies. J Neural Transm. 2005;112:1547–64.
34. Goldman SM, Tanner CM, Oakes D, Bhudhikanok GS, Gupta A, Langston JW. Head injury and Parkinson's disease risk in twins. Ann Neurol. 2006;60:65–72.
35. Hamidou B, Couratier P, Besançon C, Nicol M, Preux PM, Marin B. Epidemiological evidence that physical activity is not a risk factor for ALS. Eur J Epidemiol. 2014;29(7):459–75.
36. Harwood CA, Westgate K, Gunstone S, Brage S, Wareham NJ, McDermott CJ, et al. Long-term physical activity: an exogenous risk factor for sporadic amyotrophic lateral sclerosis? Amyotroph Lateral Scler Frontotemporal Degener. 2016;17(5–6):377–84.
37. Longstreth WT, McGuire V, Koepsell TD, Wang Y, van Belle G. Risk of amyotrophic lateral sclerosis and history of physical activity: a population-based case-control study. Arch Neurol. 1998;55(2):201.
38. Chio A, Benzi G, Dossena M, Mutani R, Mora G. Severely increased risk of amyotrophic lateral sclerosis among Italian professional football players. Brain. 2005;128(Pt 3):472–6.
39. Chio A, Calvo A, Dossena M, Ghiglione P, Mutani R, Mora G. ALS in Italian professional soccer players: the risk is still present and could be soccer-specific. Amyotroph Lateral Scler. 2009;10(4):205–9.
40. Savica R, Parisi JE, Wold LE, Josephs KA, Ahlskog JE. High school football and risk of neurodegeneration: a community-based study. Mayo Clin Proc. 2012;87(4):335–40.

41. Pupillo E, Messina P, Giussani G, Logroscino G, Zoccolella S, Chiò A, et al. Physical activity and amyotrophic lateral sclerosis: a European population-based case-control study. Ann Neurol. 2014 May;75(5):708–16.
42. Ingre C, Roos PM, Piehl F, Kamel F, Fang F. Risk factors for amyotrophic lateral sclerosis. Clin Epidemiol. 2015;7:181–93.
43. Dearborn MJ, Hastings JE. Type a personality as a mediator of stress and strain in employed women. J Hum Stress. 1982;13:53–60.
44. Orpen C. Type a personality as a moderator of the effects of role conflict, role ambiguity and role overload on individual strain. J Hum Stress. 1982;8:8–14.
45. Okamoto K, Kihira T, Kokubo Y, Kuzuhara S. Gender and age differences in lifestyle factors and risk of amyotrophic lateral sclerosis; a case-control study in Japan. J Neurol Psychol August. 2017;5:1–4.
46. Wu D, Liu B, Yin J, Xu T, Zhao S, Xu Q, et al. Detection of 8-hydroxydeoxyguanosine (8-OHdG) as a biomarker of oxidative damage in peripheral leukocyte DNA by UHPLC-MS/MS. J Chromatogr B Analyt Technol Biomed Life Sci. 2017;1064:1–6.
47. Song Y, Leonard SW, Traber MG, Ho E. Zinc deficiency affects DNA damage, oxidative stress, antioxidant defenses, and DNA repair in rats. J Nutr. 2009;139:1626–31.
48. Wu LL, Chiou CC, Chang PY, et al. Urinary 8-OHdG: a marker of oxidative stress to DNA and a risk factor for cancer, atherosclerosis and diabetics. Clin Chim Acta. 2004;339:1–9.
49. Sato S, Mizuno Y, Hattori N, et al. Urinary 8-hydroxydeoxyguanosine levels as a biomarker for progression of Parkinson disease. Neurology. 2005;64:1081–3.
50. Kihira T, Okamoto K, Sakurai I, Arakawa Y, Wakayama I, Takamiya K, et al. Nutritional status and risk of amyotrophic lateral sclerosis in Japan. Intern Med. 2017;56(12):1497–506.
51. Morimoto S, Kuzuhara S, Kokubo Y. Increased oxidative stress in patients with amyotrophic lateral sclerosis/Parkinsonism-dementia complex in the Kii peninsula, Japan. Mov Disord. 2009 Jan 15;24(1):123–6.
52. Yase Y. The pathogenesis of amyotrophic lateral sclerosis. Lancet. 1972;II:292–6.
53. Garruto RM, Yanagihara R, Gajdusek DC, Arion DM. Concentrations of heavy metals and essential minerals in garden soil and drinking water in the western Pacific. In: Chen KM, Yase Y, (eds). Amyotrophic lateral sclerosis in Asia and Oseania. National Taiwan University, Shyan-Fu Chou, 1984: 265–330.
54. Kihira T, Okamoto K, Yoshida S, et al. Environmental characteristics and oxidative stress of inhabitants and patients with amyotrophic lateral sclerosis in a high-incidence area on the Kii peninsula, Japan. Intern Med. 2013;52:1479–86.
55. Kihira T, Okamoto K, Sakurai I, Arakawa Y, Wakayama I, Takamiya K, et al. Lifestyle changes and oxidative stress in a high-incidence area of amyotrophic lateral sclerosis in the Southwestern Kii Peninsula, Japan. Intern Med. 2017;56(12):1497–506.
56. Taysi S, Cikman O, Kaya A, Demircan B, Gumustekin K, Yilmaz A, et al. Increased oxidant stress and decreased antioxidant status in erythrocytes of rats fed with zinc deficient diet. Biol Trace Elem Res. 2008;123(1–3):161–7.
57. Dobson AW, Erikson KM, Aschner M. Manganese neurotoxicity. Ann N Y Acad Sci. 2004;1012:115–28.
58. Roos PM, Lierhagen S, Flaten TP, Syversen T, Vesterberg O, Nordberg M. Manganese in cerebrospinal fluid and blood plasma of patients with amyotrophic lateral sclerosis. Exp Biol Med (Maywood). 2012;237(7):803–10.
59. Allen DA, Yaqoob MM, Harwood SM. Mechanism of high glucose-induced apoptosis and its relationship to diabetic complications. J Nutr Biochem. 2005;16:705–13.
60. Perez J, Ware MA, Chevalier S, Gougeon R, Bennett GJ, Shir Y. Dietary fat and protein interact in suppressing neuropathic pain-related disorders following a partial sciatic ligation injury in rats. Pain. 2004;111:297–305.
61. Wang ZJ, Li GM, Nie BM, Lu Y, Yin M. Neuroprotective effect of stearic acid against oxidative stress via phosphatidylinositol 3-kinase pathway. Chem Biol Interact. 2006;160:80–7.
62. Russo A, Izzo AA, Borrelli F, Renis M, Vanella A. Free radical scavenging capacity and protective effect of Bacopa monniera L. on DNA damage. Phytother Res. 2003;17(8):870–5.

63. Okamoto K. Dietary antioxidant intake and risk of an amyotrophic lateral sclerosis in Japan. J Public Health. 2017;1(2):1–5.
64. Wang H, O'Reilly ÉJ, Weisskopf MG, Logroscino G, McCullough ML, Schatzkin A, et al. Vitamin E intake and risk of amyotrophic lateral sclerosis: a pooled analysis of data from 5 prospective cohort studies. Am J Epidemiol. 2011 Mar 15;173(6):595–602.
65. Okamoto K, Kihira T, Kobashi G, Washio M, Sasaki S, Yokoyama T, et al. Fruit and vegetable intake and risk of amyotrophic lateral sclerosis in Japan. Neuroepidemiology. 2009;32(4):251–6.
66. Okamoto K. Dietary patterns and risk of amyotrophic lateral Screlosis: a case-control study in Japan. J Neurol Epidemiol. 2017. 1–6.

Chapter 5 Case-Control Study of Idiopathic Parkinson's Disease in Japan

Keiko Tanaka and Yoshihiro Miyake

Abstract The causes of Parkinson's disease (PD) still remain unclear, although a complex interaction in genetic and environmental factors is likely to be associated with the development and progression of the disease. We conducted a hospital-based case-control study named the Fukuoka Kinki Parkinson's Disease Study to examine the associations between risk and preventive factors including genetic factors and the risk of PD in Japan.

As preventive factors, we confirmed that smoking habits and caffeine intake reduce the risk of PD. Further, the "Healthy dietary pattern" which was characterized by a high intake of vegetables, seaweed, pulses, mushrooms, fruits, and fish was likely to be associated with a reduced risk of PD. *LARK2 Gly2385Arg, MAOB, COMT, SNCA, UCHL1S18Y, PARK16, VDR, APOE* SNPs were associated with the risk of PD. There were no associations between *GST*, *BST1,* or *MDR1* and the risk of PD.

In order to establish evidence on various factors for PD in Japanese, further studies with a large number of subjects are needed.

Keywords Case-control studies · Diet · Environmental factors · Occupation · Parkinson's disease · Risk · SNPs

5.1 Introduction

Parkinson's disease (PD) is a chronic, movement-related disease of adults and the second most common neurodegenerative disease after Alzheimer's disease [1, 2]. As the age increases, the prevalence of PD is rising. According to the patient survey in Japan at 2014, the number of patients of PD was estimated 163 thousand.

K. Tanaka (✉) · Y. Miyake
Department of Epidemiology and Preventive Medicine, Ehime University Graduate School of Medicine, Ehime, Japan
e-mail: tanaka.keiko.jn@ehime-u.ac.jp

M. Washio, G. Kobashi (eds.), *Epidemiological Studies of Specified Rare and Intractable Disease*, Current Topics in Environmental Health and Preventive Medicine, https://doi.org/10.1007/978-981-13-1096-6_5

The causes of PD still remain unclear, although a complex interaction in genetic and environmental factors is likely to be associated with the development and progression of the disease. The diagnosis is made clinically; however, there is the potential for confusion with other disorders with prominent symptoms and signs of parkinsonism such as postencephalitic, drug-induced, and arteriosclerotic parkinsonism [1]. Risk and preventive factors of PD have been investigated in past decades worldwide. On the other hand, evidence for related factors of PD was very limited in Japan. For example, smoking is widely accepted as one of the potential protective factors of PD; however, in Japan, only one study investigated the association between smoking and the risk of PD [3].

In this chapter, using data from a case-control study of PD among Japanese named the Fukuoka Kinki Parkinson's Disease Study, risk and preventive factors of PD were reviewed.

5.2 The Fukuoka Kinki Parkinson's Disease Study

5.2.1 Study Population

PD cases were recruited at three university hospitals and one national hospital in Fukuoka Prefecture, and at three university hospitals, three national hospitals, and one municipal hospital in Osaka, Kyoto, and Wakayama Prefectures. Eligible cases were patients who were within 6 years of the onset of PD and who had been diagnosed by one of the collaborating neurologists at one of the 11 collaborating hospitals according to the United Kingdom PD Society Brain Bank clinical diagnostic criteria [4]. The neurologists in charge asked their eligible PD patients to participate in the case-control study. Of 298 eligible PD cases identified during the period between April 1, 2006 and March 31, 2008, 250 agreed to participate in the study (response rate: 84%).

In the same time period, control subjects were recruited from departments other than neurology (orthopedic surgery, ophthalmology, otorhinolaryngology, plastic surgery, and oral surgery) at three of the 11 collaborating hospitals: one university hospital in Fukuoka Prefecture and one university hospital in Osaka and one national hospital in Kyoto. Control subjects were not matched to cases, either individually or in larger groups. Control candidates, who were inpatients or outpatients without neurodegenerative diseases at any of these three hospitals, were approached by an attending doctor or by one of our research nurses to participate in the case-control study. Eventually, 372 control candidates participated in our study whereas 156 refused (response rate: 70%).

Of the 250 cases and 372 control subjects who participated in our study, 240 cases and 371 controls gave informed consent to genotyping. In the study of genetic polymorphisms, excluded were 11 cases and 12 controls with a family history of PD.

The ethics committees of the 11 collaborating hospitals (Fukuoka University, Utano National Hospital, Osaka City University, Kyushu University, Wakayama Medical University, Kyoto University, Kurume University, Minami-Kyoto National Hospital, Toneyama National Hospital, Kyoto City Hospital, and National Omuta Hospital) approved our case-control study. Written informed consent was obtained from all subjects.

5.2.2 *Measurement*

Participants filled out a set of two self-administered questionnaires and mailed these materials to the data management center or handed them to research nurses. Our research technicians completed missing answers and/or illogical data by telephone or in-person interview.

One of the self-administered questionnaires elicited information on age, sex, educational levels, type of job held for the longest period of time, exposure to 13 specific occupational agents, smoking habits, passive smoking exposure at home and at work, leisure-time exercise, and a history of disorders.

A second questionnaire was a validated self-administered, semiquantitative, comprehensive diet history questionnaire (DHQ) that was used to assess dietary habits during the preceding month [5, 6]. Estimates of daily intake of foods (150 items in total), energy, and selected nutrients were calculated using an ad hoc computer algorithm for the DHQ based on the Standard Tables of Food Composition in Japan [7, 8]. Energy-adjusted intake by the residual method was used for the analyses [9]. Intake of foods and nutrients was categorized at quartile points based on the distribution of intake among control subjects.

5.2.3 *DNA Extraction and Genotyping*

Genomic DNA from buccal specimens collected with BuccalAmp swabs (Epicenter BioTechnologies, Madison, WI, USA) was extracted using a QIAmp DNA mini kit (Qiagen, Inc., Valencia, CA, USA). Selected SNPs were genotyped using TaqMan SNP Genotyping Assays on the StepOnePlus machine (Applied Biosystems, Foster City, CA, USA) according to the manufacturer's instructions.

5.2.4 *Statistical Analysis*

Multiple logistic regression analysis was used to estimate the adjusted odds ratios (ORs) and 95% confidence intervals (CIs) of PD for factors under study.

5.3 Results

5.3.1 Characteristics

The characteristics of cases and controls are shown in Table 5.1. Compared with control subjects, cases were more likely to be old and thin and to report never having smoked (Table 5.1). There were no differences between cases and controls with regard to sex, region of residence, and education. Dairy intake of foods and nutrients of subjects is shown in Table 5.2.

5.3.2 Smoking Habits and Occupational Factors

Table 5.3 shows adjusted OR and 95% CI for PD in relation to smoking habits [3] and occupational factors [10]. Ever smoking was associated with a reduced risk of PD. Risk for former smokers was intermediate between the high risk for never smokers and the low risk for current smokers. However, no significant association was detected for passive smoking at home or at work (data not shown).

In analyses of occupational factors, jobs held for the longest period of time were coded using the Japanese Standard Occupational Classification and stratified into 11 major groups (professional and technical; managers and officials; clerical and related fields; sales; service; protective service; farming, fishing and forestry; transport and communication; production; materials handling; and construction and extraction). The mean duration of the job held for the longest time in the study population was 24.8 years. Occupational exposure to agent was defined as present if the subject had been exposed to any of 10 specific occupational agents (metal,

Table 5.1 Characteristics of study population

	n (%) or mean (SD)		
Variable	Cases (*n* = 249)	Controls (*n* = 368)	*P*-value
Sex (% male)	93 (37.4)	141 (38.3)	0.81
Age (years)	68.5 (8.6)	66.6 (8.5)	0.006
Region of residence (%)			0.13
Fukuoka	89 (35.7)	154 (41.9)	
Kinki	160 (64.3)	214 (58.2)	
Educational level (%)			0.81
<10	51 (20.5)	77 (20.9)	
10-12	122 (49.0)	171 (46.5)	
13+	76 (30.5)	120 (32.6)	
Body mass index (kg/m^2)	22.3 (3.3)	23.0 (3.4)	0.01
Pack-years of smoking (%)			0.0004
Never	185 (74.3)	222 (60.3)	
0<-29.9	37 (14.9)	65 (17.7)	
30.0+	27 (10.8)	81 (22.0)	

Table 5.2 Daily intake[a] of nutrients and foods of the study population

	n (%) or mean (SD)	
Variable	Cases (*n* = 249)	Controls (*n* = 368)
Total energy (kJ)	8435.4 (2636.8)	8348.8 (3067.7)
Coffee (g)	119.0 (138.8)	172.7 (207.7)
Black tea (g)	23.8 (95.3)	27.8 (81.5)
Japanese and Chinese teas (g)	507.2 (407.1)	591.8 (453.0)
Total vegetables (g)	270.6 (149.4)	276.1 (181.9)
Green and yellow vegetables (g)	102.2 (64.8)	106.0 (84.8)
Other vegetables (g)	168.4 (110.6)	170.1 (132.3)
Total fruit (g)	180.7 (136.5)	166.5 (141.9)
Milk (g)	91.9 (85.7)	95.5 (103.4)
Yogurt (g)	36.6 (45.7)	38.0 (52.4)
Cheese (g)	3.6 (6.7)	4.1 (9.4)
Ice cream (g)	16.8 (29.1)	16.1 (29.5)
Caffeine (mg)	287.2 (193.8)	358.7 (224.0)
Calcium (mg)	553.8 (185.5)	556.6 (219.9)
Vitamin C (mg)	127.1 (64.2)	119.3 (70.2)
Vitamin E (mg)	8.6 (2.4)	8.4 (2.9)
α-Carotene (μg)	327.2 (314.1)	335.2 (339.2)
β-Carotene (μg)	3021.7 (1630.9)	3126.0 (2024.7)
Vitamin D (μg)	10.9 (6.4)	10.0 (5.7)
Vitamin B_6 (mg)	1.3 (0.4)	1.3 (0.4)
Dietary glycemic index	65.1 (4.7)	65.4 (5.3)
Iron (mg)	7.5 (1.9)	7.6 (2.2)
Magnesium (mg)	266.8 (63.5)	274.4 (71.0)
Zinc (μg)	8.3 (1.5)	8.1 (1.4)
Copper (μg)	1.2 (0.2)	1.2 (0.2)
Manganese (mg)	4.1 (1.3)	4.4 (1.5)
Total fat (g)	57.9 (13.7)	56.3 (17.2)
Saturated fatty acids (g)	15.6 (4.6)	15.2 (5.7)
Monounsaturated fatty acids (g)	19.9 (5.6)	19.3 (6.6)
n-3 polyunsaturated fatty acids (g)	2.9 (1.1)	2.8 (1.2)
α-Linolenic acid (g)	1.6 (0.6)	1.6 (0.7)
Eicosapentaenoic acid (g)	0.37 (0.25)	0.35 (0.25)
Docosahexaenoic acid (g)	0.60 (0.38)	0.56 (0.39)
n-6 Polyunsaturated fatty acids (g)	10.5 (3.0)	10.4 (3.4)
Linoleic acid (g)	10.2 (3.0)	10.2 (3.4)
Arachidonic acid (g)	0.15 (0.05)	0.14 (0.06)
Cholesterol (mg)	331.3 (129.5)	300.9 (132.5)
Alcohol (g)	5.5 (15.5)	10.0 (25.8)

[a]Nutrient intake was adjusted for total energy intake using the residual method except for the dietary glycemic index

Table 5.3 Adjusted odds ratios for PD in relation to smoking habits and occupational factors

Factor	*n* (%)		Adjusted odds ratio[a]	95% confidence interval
	Cases (*n* = 249)	Controls (*n* = 369)		
Smoking status[a]				
No	185 (74.3)	222 (60.2)	1.00	
Yes	64 (25.7)	147 (39.8)	0.38	0.24 to 0.60
Cigarette smoking[a]				
Never	185 (74.3)	222 (60.2)	1.00	
Former	57 (22.9)	96 (26.0)	0.51	0.32 to 0.82
Current	7 (2.8)	51 (13.8)	0.12	0.05 to 0.27
Pack-years of smoking[a]				
None	185 (74.3)	222 (60.2)	1.00	
0 < −29.9	37 (14.9)	65 (17.6)	0.50	0.29 to 0.83
30.0+	27 (10.8)	82 (22.2)	0.28	0.15 to 0.49
Job held for the longest period of time[b]				
Professional or technical	20 (8.0)	45 (12.2)	0.59	0.32 to 1.06
Manager or official	36 (14.5)	47 (12.7)	1.20	0.69 to 2.06
Clerical or related occupation	63 (25.3)	76 (20.6)	1.36	0.91 to 2.04
Sales	19 (7.6)	36 (9.8)	0.87	0.47 to 1.56
Service	12 (4.8)	22 (6.0)	0.80	0.37 to 1.67
Protective service	4 (1.6)	3 (0.8)	2.73	0.56 to 14.86
Farming, fishing, or forestry	11 (4.4)	16 (4.3)	0.95	0.41 to 2.15
Transport or communication	10 (4.0)	9 (2.4)	1.74	0.65 to 4.74
Production	39 (15.7)	48 (13.0)	1.11	0.68 to 1.81
Materials handling	0 (0.0)	2 (0.5)	–	–
Construction or extraction	14 (5.6)	21 (5.7)	1.25	0.59 to 2.60
Occupational agents[b]				
Any	36 (14.5)	61 (16.5)	0.90	0.56 to 1.43
Metal	6 (2.4)	7 (1.9)	1.26	0.38 to 4.01
Wood	5 (2.0)	10 (2.7)	0.95	0.28 to 2.89
Asbestos	1 (0.4)	7 (1.9)	0.23	0.01 to 1.40
Coal	2 (0.8)	2 (0.5)	1.02	0.12 to 8.97
Stone or sand	4 (1.6)	3 (0.8)	1.98	0.39 to 11.18
Solvents	7 (2.8)	12 (3.3)	1.10	0.38 to 2.95
Chalk	5 (2.0)	6 (1.6)	1.18	0.32 to 4.18
Pesticides	15 (6.0)	28 (7.6)	0.75	0.37 to 1.46
Herbicides	12 (4.8)	19 (5.2)	0.87	0.39 to 1.88
Fungicides	7 (2.8)	12 (3.3)	0.94	0.34 to 2.47

[a]Adjusted for age, sex, region of residence, educational level, and occupational exposure.
[b]Adjusted for age, sex, region of residence, educational level, and pack-years of smoking.

wood, asbestos, coal, stone and sand, solvents, chalk, pesticide, herbicides, or fungicides) for 10 or more hours per week for more than 1 year. None of the occupational groups was related to the risk of PD. According to a stratified analysis by sex, the decrease risk of PD for persons in professional or technical occupations was statistically significant only among men. Regarding exposure to occupational agents, there was no statistical significance concerning exposure to any of the occupational agents and the risk of PD, although roughly a twofold increases in OR was observed for exposure to stone or sand.

5.3.3 Hypertension, Hypercholesterolemia, and Diabetes

Table 5.4 shows adjusted OR and 95% CI for PD in relation to vascular risk factors [11]. Hypertension, hypercholesterolemia, and diabetes mellitus were defined as being present when cases had received antihypertensive, cholesterol lowering, and diabetic medications, respectively, prior to the onset of PD or when controls had received such medications at the time of answering the questionnaires. Hypertension, hypercholesterolemia, and diabetes mellitus were significantly associated with decreased risk of PD. No significant differences were observed in the association between vascular risk factors and the risk of PD among men and women.

5.3.4 Diet

5.3.4.1 Alcohol and Caffeine

Alcohol intake during peak drinking period was not associated with the risk of PD (data not shown) [12]. However, when we assessed daily ethanol intake separately for each type of alcohol, only Japanese sake (rice wine) was significantly associated with an increased risk of PD (Table 5.5).

Table 5.4 Adjusted odds ratios for PD in relation to a history of disorders

Factor	n (%)			
	Cases (*n* = 249)	Controls (*n* = 368)	Adjusted odds ratio[a]	95% confidence interval
Hypertension				
No	190 (76.3)	225 (61.1)	1.00	
Yes	59 (23.7)	143 (38.9)	0.43	0.29 to 0.64
Hypercholesterolemia				
No	225 (90.4)	307 (83.4)	1.00	
Yes	24 (9.6)	61 (16.6)	0.58	0.33 to 0.97
Diabetes mellitus				
No	239 (96.0)	329 (89.4)	1.00	
Yes	10 (4.0)	39 (10.6)	0.38	0.17 to 0.79

[a]Adjusted for age, sex, region of residence, pack-years of smoking, educational level, leisure-time exercise, body mass index, dietary intake of energy, cholesterol, vitamin E, alcohol, and coffee and the dietary glycemic index

Table 5.5 Adjusted odds ratios for PD according to alcohol drinking amount per day during "peak" period for types of alcohol

Alcohol drinking amount per day during "peak" period (ethanol, g)	*n* (%) Cases (*n* = 214)	Controls (*n* = 327)	Adjusted odds ratio[a]	95% confidence interval
Beer				
Nondrinker	127 (59.4)	195 (59.6)	1.00	
0.1–65.9	75 (35.1)	121 (37.0)	0.99	0.61 to 1.59
≥ 66.0	12 (5.6)	11 (3.4)	2.13	0.80 to 5.82
P for trend			0.39	
Japanese sake (rice wine)				
Nondrinker	146 (68.2)	261 (79.8)	1.00	
0.1–65.9	58 (27.1)	59 (18.0)	2.27	1.34 to 3.89
≥ 66.0	10 (4.7)	7 (2.1)	3.39	1.10 to 11.0
P for trend			0.001	
Shochu (a distilled alcoholic beverage made in Japan)				
Nondrinker	180 (84.1)	273 (83.5)	1.00	
0.1–65.9	18 (8.4)	32 (9.8)	1.01	0.50 to 1.98
≥ 66.0	16 (7.5)	22 (6.7)	1.29	0.59 to 2.78
P for trend			0.58	
Wine				
Nondrinker	187 (87.4)	294 (89.9)	1.00	
0.1–65.9	24 (11.2)	32 (9.8)	1.06	0.57 to 1.95
≥ 66.0	3 (1.4)	1 (0.3)	6.11	0.67 to 1.34
P for trend			0.36	
Whisky				
Nondrinker	177 (82.7)	283 (86.5)	1.00	
0.1–65.9	30 (14.0)	38 (11.6)	1.60	0.88 to 2.93
≥ 66.0	7 (3.3)	6 (1.8)	2.25	0.67 to 7.83
P for trend			0.06	

[a]Adjusted for age, sex, region of residence, pack-years of smoking, educational level, body mass index, alcohol flushing status, presence of medication history for hypertension, hypercholesterolemia and diabetes, dietary intake of caffeine, cholesterol, vitamin E, vitamin B6, and dietary glycemic index

Intake of coffee, black tea, and Japanese and Chinese teas was significantly inversely associated with the risk of PD (Table 5.6) [13]. A clear dose-response relationship was observed between total caffeine intake and the risk of PD.

5.3.4.2 Foods and Nutrients

Tables 5.7 and 5.8 show adjusted ORs for associations between intake of vegetables, fruits, and antioxidant vitamins and the risk of PD [14]. Consumption of green and yellow vegetables in the third quartile, but not the second and fourth quartiles,

Table 5.6 Adjusted odds ratios for PD according to intake of coffee, black tea, and Japanese and Chinese teas and caffeine

Variables[b]	No of cases/control subjects	Adjusted odds ratio[a]	95% confidence interval
Coffee			
Q1 (< 26)	76/92	1.00	
Q2 (26 to <122)	73/92	0.92	0.58 to 1.44
Q3 (122 to <243)	65/92	0.80	0.50 to 1.28
Q4 (243 ≤)	35/92	0.52	0.52 to 0.90
P for trend		0.02	
Black tea			
Q1 (< −0.5)	67/92	1.00	
Q2 (−0.5 to <8.7)	84/92	1.13	0.71 to 1.82
Q3 (8.7 to <20.8)	49/92	0.61	0.36 to 1.02
Q4 (20.8 ≤)	49/92	0.58	0.35 to 0.97
P for trend		0.005	
Japanese and Chinese teas			
Q1 (< 295)	84/92	1.00	
Q2 (295 to <492)	56/92	0.63	0.39 to 1.02
Q3 (492 to <840)	64/92	0.73	0.45 to 1.18
Q4 (840 ≤)	45/92	0.59	0.35 to 0.995
P for trend		0.08	
Caffeine			
Q1 (<194)	88/92	1.00	
Q2 (194 to <315)	70/92	0.76	0.48 to 1.21
Q3 (315 to <496)	55/92	0.64	0.40 to 1.04
Q4 (496 ≤)	36/92	0.46	0.46 to 0.78
P for trend		0.003	

[a]Adjusted for age, sex, region of residence, pack-years of smoking, educational level, body mass index, alcohol flushing status, presence of medication history for hypertension, hypercholesterolemia and diabetes, dietary intake of caffeine, cholesterol, vitamin E, vitamin B6, and dietary glycemic index

[b]Quartile were based on intake in g/day (except for caffeine: mg/day) adjusted for energy intake using residual methods

was independently associated with a decreased risk of PD; however, the inverse linear trend was not significant in the multivariate model. There were no evident associations between intake of total vegetables, vegetables other than green and yellow vegetables, or total fruit and PD. On the other hand, higher consumption of vitamin E and β-carotene was significantly associated with a reduced risk of PD.

Table 5.9 shows adjusted ORs for associations between intake of dairy products, calcium, and vitamin D and the risk of PD [15]. Total dairy product consumption was not materially associated with the risk of PD. No evident relationships were observed between intake of milk, yogurt, cheese, or ice cream and the risk of PD. There were no measurable associations between consumption of calcium or

Table 5.7 Adjusted odds ratios for PD by quartiles of intake of vegetables and fruits

Variables[b]	No of cases/control subjects	Adjusted odds ratio[a]	95% confidence interval
Total vegetables			
Q1 (<175.5)	62/92	1.00	
Q2 (175.5 to <246.6)	70/92	0.81	0.49 to 1.32
Q3 (246.6 to <346.2)	61/92	0.70	0.42 to 1.16
Q4 (346.2 ≤)	56/92	0.69	0.40 to 1.16
P for trend		0.14	
Green and yellow vegetables			
Q1 (< 61.1)	71/92	1.00	
Q2 (61.1 to <92.9)	58/92	0.64	0.39 to 1.03
Q3 (92.9 to <131.7)	54/92	0.56	0.34 to 0.93
Q4 (131.7 ≤)	66/92	0.66	0.40 to 1.08
P for trend		0.10	
Other vegetables			
Q1 (< 101.1)	57/92	1.00	
Q2 (101.1 to <148.05)	75/92	1.10	0.68 to 1.79
Q3 (148.05 to <210.9)	64/92	0.90	0.54 to 1.49
Q4 (210.9 ≤)	53/92	0.78	0.46 to 1.33
P for trend		0.25	
Total fruit			
Q1 (< 86.8)	56/92	1.00	
Q2 (86.8 to <138.2)	56/92	0.94	0.57 to 1.57
Q3 (138.2 to <225.7)	69/92	0.98	0.59 to 1.64
Q4 (225.7 ≤)	68/92	0.97	0.57 to 1.65
P for trend		0.96	

[a]Adjusted for age, sex, region of residence, pack-years of smoking, educational level, body mass index, dietary intake of cholesterol, alcohol, total dairy products, and coffee and the dietary glycemic index

[b]Quartile were based on intake in g/day adjusted for energy intake using residual methods

vitamin D and PD. No significant interactions were observed between the dietary exposures and sex regarding PD.

Higher intake of iron, magnesium, and zinc was independently associated with a reduced risk of PD (Table 5.10) [16]. There were no relationships between the intake of copper or manganese and the risk of PD. Additional adjustment for intake of magnesium, zinc, and copper as continuous variables did not materially alter the significant inverse relationship between iron consumption and the risk of PD (data not shown). After further adjustment for intake of iron, zinc, and copper, the significant inverse association between magnesium intake and PD remained, the OR

Table 5.8 Adjusted odds ratios for PD by quartiles of intake of antioxidant vitamins

Variables[b]	No of cases/control subjects	Adjusted odds ratio[a]	95% confidence interval
Vitamin C			
Q1 (< 84.7)	60/92	1.00	
Q2 (84.7 to <109.6)	52/92	0.71	0.43 to 1.19
Q3 (109.6 to <147.7)	64/92	0.82	0.49 to 1.37
Q4 (147.7 ≤)	73/92	0.92	0.54 to 1.55
P for trend		0.95	
Vitamin E			
Q1 (<7.19)	73/92	1.00	
Q2 (7.19 to <8.44)	55/92	0.49	0.29 to 0.81
Q3 (8.44 to <9.759)	54/92	0.41	0.24 to 0.71
Q4 (9.759 ≤)	67/92	0.45	0.25 to 0.79
P for trend		0.009	
α-Carotene			
Q1 (<137.5)	68/92	1.00	
Q2 (137.5 to <262.6)	60/92	0.71	0.43 to 1.15
Q3 (262.6 to <504.3)	66/92	0.69	0.42 to 1.13
Q4 (504.3 ≤)	55/92	0.61	0.36 to 1.02
P for trend		0.08	
β-Carotene			
Q1 (< 1836.1)	63/92	1.00	
Q2 (1836.1 to <2906.4)	42/92	0.80	0.48 to 1.31
Q3 (2906.4 to <4080.9)	50/92	0.64	0.38 to 1.08
Q4 (4080.9 ≤)	94/92	0.56	0.33 to 0.97
P for trend		0.03	
Cryptoxanthin			
Q1 (<115.0)	63/92	1.00	
Q2 (115.0 to <242.0)	42/92	0.52	0.30 to 0.87
Q3 (242.0 to <429.0)	50/92	0.60	0.35 to 1.003
Q4 (429.0 ≤)	94/92	1.16	0.71 to 1.89
P for trend		0.30	

[a]Adjusted for age, sex, region of residence, pack-years of smoking, educational level, body mass index, dietary intake of cholesterol, alcohol, total dairy products, and coffee and the dietary glycemic index

[b]Quartile were based on intake in μg/day (except for vitamins C and E: mg/day) for adjusted for energy intake using residual methods

between extreme quartiles being 0.33 (95% CI: 0.13–0.81, *P* for trend = 0.007). When intake of iron, magnesium, and copper was further adjusted, the inverse exposure-response relationship between zinc intake and PD fell just short of the level of significance although the further adjusted OR between extreme quartiles was significant at 0.50 (95% CI, 0.26–0.95, *P* for trend = 0.055). The inverse association

Table 5.9 Adjusted odds ratios for PD by quartiles of intake of dairy products, calcium and vitamin D

Variables[b]	No of cases/control subjects	Adjusted odds ratio[a]	95% confidence interval
Total dairy products			
Q1 (< 58.7)	57/92	1.00	
Q2 (58.7 to <132.5)	59/92	1.01	0.61 to 1.67
Q3 (132.5 to <208.4)	69/92	1.07	0.64 to 1.77
Q4 (208.4 ≤)	64/92	0.85	0.50 to 1.45
P for trend		0.62	
Milk			
Q1 (<18.2)	65/92	1.00	
Q2 (18.2 to <68.5)	57/92	0.80	0.48 to 1.33
Q3 (68.5 to <149.3)	48/92	0.62	0.36 to 1.04
Q4 (149.3 ≤)	79/92	0.96	0.59 to 1.58
P for trend		0.75	
Yogurt			
Q1 (<2.57)	66/92	1.00	0.42 to 1.16
Q2 (2.57 to <11.5)	50/92	0.70	0.63 to 1.75
Q3 (11.5 to <72.6)	70/92	1.05	0.47 to 1.31
Q4 (72.6 ≤)	63/92	0.63	
P for trend			
Cheese			
Q1 (< 0.226)	65/92	1.00	
Q2 (0.226 to <1.44)	72/92	1.26	0.77 to 2.05
Q3 (1.44 to <3.91)	48/92	0.82	0.49 to 1.39
Q4 (3.91 ≤)	64/92	0.99	0.61 to 1.62
P for trend		0.59	
Ice cream			
Q1 (< 2.01)	68/92	1.00	
Q2 (2.01 to <8.65)	67/92	0.98	0.61 to 1.59
Q3 (8.65 to <18.13)	50/92	0.72	0.43 to 1.20
Q4 (18.13 ≤)	64/92	0.85	0.51 to 1.40
P for trend		0.35	
Calcium			
Q1 (< 421.6)	61/92	1.00	
Q2 (421.6 to <539.8)	59/92	0.77	0.46 to 1.29
Q3 (539.8 to <669.2)	70/92	0.87	0.50 to 1.49
Q4 (669.2 ≤)	59/92	0.69	0.37 to 1.30
P for trend		0.37	
Vitamin D			
Q1 (< 7.129)	66/92	1.00	
Q2 (7.129 to <9.30)	47/92	0.65	0.38 to 1.09
Q3 (9.30 to <12.82)	69/92	0.83	0.50 to 1.37

Table 5.9 (continued)

Variables[b]	No of cases/control subjects	Adjusted odds ratio[a]	95% confidence interval
Q4 (12.82 ≤)	67/92	0.82	0.46 to 1.47
P for trend		0.69	

[a]Adjusted for age, sex, region of residence, pack-years of smoking, educational level, body mass index, dietary intake of cholesterol, vitamin E, β-Carotene, vitamin B6 caffeine, iron, alcohol, and the dietary glycemic index

[b]Quartile were based on intake in g/day (except for calcium: mg/day and vitamin D: μg/day) for adjusted for energy intake using residual methods

between copper intake and PD had completely disappeared after further adjustment for intake of iron, magnesium, and zinc.

Compared with arachidonic acid intake in the first quartile, consumption of that in the fourth quartile was significantly related to an increased risk of PD (Table 5.11) [17]. Cholesterol intake was also significantly positively associated with the risk of PD. On the other hand, there was no association between consumption of total fat, saturated fatty acids, monounsaturated fatty acids, n-3 polyunsaturated fatty acids, α-linolenic acid, eicosapentaenoic acid, docosahexaenoic acid, n-6 polyunsaturated fatty acids, and linoleic acid or the ratio of n-3 to n-6 polyunsaturated fatty acid intake and the risk of PD.

5.3.4.3 Glycemic Index and Dietary Pattern

Glycemic index was significantly inversely associated with the risk of PD [18]: multivariate ORs, by adjusting for potential confounding factors, including sex, age, region, pack-years of smoking, education, body mass index, and intake of fat, vitamin E, iron, and alcohol (95% CIs), for PD in the first, second, third, and forth quartiles dietary glycemic index were 1.00 (reference), 1.03 (0.64–1.66), 0.68 (0.41–1.15), and 0.61 (0.34–1.09), respectively (P for trend = 0.04). Conversely, no significant associations were observed for other dietary carbohydrates, including available carbohydrate intake (P for trend = 0.28), dietary fiber intake (P for trend = 0.73), or dietary GL (P for trend = 0.77).

In this study subjects, three dietary patterns were identified [19]. Factor 1, which loaded heavily on green and yellow vegetables, seaweed, pulses, other vegetables, mushrooms, potatoes, fruits, fish, sea products, miso soup, Japanese and Chinese tea, and low intake of alcoholic beverages, was labelled the "Healthy pattern." Factor 2, which had high loadings for beef and pork, chicken, vegetable oil, shellfish, processed meat, salt-containing seasonings, and eggs, was labelled the "Western pattern." Factor 3, which had high loadings for bread, confectionaries, dairy products, sugar, black tea, fruit and vegetable juices, coffee and cocoa, butter, noodles, and soft drinks, was labelled the "Light meal" pattern. After adjustment for sex, age, region of residence, pack-years of smoking, educational level, and body mass index, multivariate OR (95% CI) for PD in the highest quartile of the Health pattern was 0.54 (0.32 to 0.92) compared with the lowest quartile. No associations with PD were detected for the other two dietary patterns.

Table 5.10 Adjusted odds ratios for PD by quartiles of intake of metals

Variables[b]	No of cases/control subjects	Adjusted odds ratio[a]	95% confidence interval
Iron			
Q1 (< 6.42)	71/92	1.00	
Q2 (6.42 to <7.63)	80/92	0.70	0.41 to 1.18
Q3 (7.63 to <8.73)	51/92	0.30	0.18 to 0.63
Q4 (8.73 ≤)	47/92	0.26	0.12 to 0.55
P for trend		<0.0001	
Magnesium			
Q1 (< 234.2)	79/92	1.00	
Q2 (234.2 to <269.8)	69/92	0.64	0.38 to 1.06
Q3 (269.8 to <312.9)	51/92	0.40	0.22 to 0.73
Q4 (312.9 ≤)	50/92	0.33	0.15 to 0.71
P for trend		0.002	
Zinc			
Q1 (< 7.53)	69/92	1.00	
Q2 (7.53 to <8.13)	56/92	0.54	0.32 to 0.90
Q3 (8.13 to <8.90)	63/92	0.52	0.30 to 0.90
Q4 (8.90 ≤)	61/92	0.43	0.23 to 0.80
P for trend		0.01	
Copper			
Q1 (< 1.10)	78/92	1.00	
Q2 (1.10 to <1.208)	60/92	0.68	0.41 to 1.12
Q3 (1.208 to <1.34)	54/92	0.52	0.30 to 0.87
Q4 (1.34 ≤)	57/92	0.55	0.31 to 0.99
P for trend		0.03	
Manganese			
Q1 (< 3.32)	78/92	1.00	
Q2 (3.32 to <4.20)	67/92	0.87	0.53 to 1.43
Q3 (4.20 to <5.45)	62/92	1.06	0.60 to 1.87
Q4 (5.45 ≤)	42/92	0.92	0.45 to 1.87
P for trend		0.98	

[a]Adjusted for age, sex, region of residence, pack-years of smoking, educational level, body mass index, dietary intake of cholesterol, vitamin E, β-Carotene, vitamin B6 caffeine, alcohol, and the dietary glycemic index

[b]Quartile were based on intake in mg/day for adjusted for energy intake using residual methods

5.3.5 *Genetic Factors*

In the present case-control study, we analyzed the associations between some single nucleotide polymorphisms (SNPs) and the risk of PD [20–29]. Table 5.12 shows the observed results of significant associations between SNPs and the risk of PD. The distributions of all examined SNPs among controls were consistent with the Hardy-Weinberg equilibrium.

Table 5.11 Adjusted odds ratios for PD by quartiles of intake of specific types of dietary fat

Variables[b]	No of cases/control subjects	Adjusted odds ratio[a]	95% confidence interval
Total fat			
Q1 (<49.5)	54/92	1.00	
Q2 (49.5 to <57.23)	62/92	1.00	0.59 to 1.67
Q3 (57.23 to <64.98)	74/92	1.21	0.72 to 2.05
Q4 (64.98 ≤)	59/92	0.95	0.52 to 1.72
P for trend		1.00	
Saturated fatty acids			
Q1 (< 12.24)	46/92	1.00	
Q2 (12.24 to <15.04)	70/92	1.36	0.82 to 2.29
Q3 (15.04 to < 18.00)	76/92	0.50	0.90 to 2.51
Q4 (18.00 ≤)	57/92	1.05	0.61 to 1.83
P for trend		0.92	
Monounsaturated fatty acids			
Q1 (<16.46)	63/92	1.00	
Q2 (16.46 to <19.35)	60/92	0.84	0.51 to 1.38
Q3 (19.35 to <22.60)	58/92	0.78	0.47 to 1.32
Q4 (22.60 ≤)	68/92	1.01	0.58 to 1.78
P for trend		0.90	
n-3 polyunsaturated fatty acids			
Q1 (< 2.258)	61/92	1.00	
Q2 (2.258 to <2.780)	71/92	1.07	0.66 to 1.75
Q3 (2.780 to <3.248)	57/92	0.92	0.55 to 1.56
Q4 (3.248 ≤)	60/92	0.93	0.52 to 1.65
P for trend		0.67	
α-Linolenic acid			
Q1 (<1.27839)	66/92	1.00	
Q2 (1.27839 to <1.5897)	64/92	0.84	0.51 to 1.38
Q3 (1.5897 to <1.880)	49/92	0.66	0.39 to 1.14
Q4 (1.880 ≤)	70/92	1.01	0.58 to 1.76
P for trend		0.95	
Eicosapentaenoic acid			
Q1 (< 0.232)	64/92	1.00	
Q2 (0.232 to <0.3155)	59/92	0.79	0.48 to 1.29
Q3 (0.3155 to <0.4708)	67/92	0.92	0.57 to 1.48
Q4 (0.4708 ≤)	59/92	0.89	0.53 to 1.50
P for trend		0.90	
Docosahexaenoic acid			
Q1 (< 0.370)	56/92	1.00	
Q2 (0.370 to <0.522)	66/92	1.02	0.63 to 1.67

(continued)

Table 5.11 (continued)

Variables[b]	No of cases/control subjects	Adjusted odds ratio[a]	95% confidence interval
Q3 (0.522 to <0.727)	62/92	1.00	0.61 to 1.65
Q4 (0.727 ≤)	65/92	1.14	0.68 to 1.93
P for trend		0.62	
n-6 polyunsaturated fatty acids			
Q1 (< 8.78)	66/92	1.00	
Q2 (8.78 to <10.27)	59	0.77	0.46 to 1.27
Q3 (1.027 to <12.25)	58/92	0.80	0.47 to 1.36
Q4 (12.25 ≤)	66/92	0.99	0.56 to 1.74
P for trend		0.92	
Linoleic acid			
Q1 (< 8.54)	65/92	1.00	
Q2 (8.54 to <10.04)	63/92	0.84	0.51 to 1.39
Q3 (10.04 to <11.938)	54/92	0.77	0.45 to 1.31
Q4 (11.938 ≤)	67/92	1.04	0.59 to 1.84
P for trend		0.86	
Arachidonic acid			
Q1 (< 0.1063)	44/92	1.00	
Q2 (0.1063 to <0.136)	62/92	1.36	0.82 to 2.29
Q3 (0.136 to <0.171)	64/92	1.48	0.87 to 2.53
Q4 (0.171 ≤)	7992	2.09	1.21 to 3.64
P for trend		0.008	
n-3/n-6 Polyunsaturated fatty acid ratio			
Q1 (<0.2139)	60/92	1.00	
Q2 (0.2139 to <0.250)	49/92	0.75	0.45 to 1.24
Q3 (0.250 to <0.306)	78/92	1.26	0.78 to 2.04
Q4 (0.306 ≤)	62/92	1.01	0.62 to 1.65
P for trend		0.51	
Cholesterol			
Q1 (< 227.8)	48/92	1.00	
Q2 (227.8 to <290.0)	51/92	0.99	0.59 to 1.68
Q3 (290.0 to <374.0)	70/92	1.42	0.85 to 2.37
Q4 (374.0 ≤)	80/92	1.78	1.04 to 3.05
P for trend		0.01	

[a]Adjusted for age, sex, region of residence, pack-years of smoking, educational level, body mass index, dietary intake of vitamin E, iron, and alcohol.
[b]Quartile were based on intake in g/day (except for cholesterol: mg/day) for adjusted for energy intake using residual methods, except for quartiles for the ratio of n-3 to n-6 polyunsaturated fatty acids, which were based on crude intake in g/day.

Monoamine oxidase B (MAOB) is one of the primary enzymes regulating metabolism of neurotransmitters such as dopamine. Because the G allele of *MAOB* rs1799836 polymorphism is associated with lower activity of brain MAOB activity, the G allele may be involved in PD susceptibility. In the present case-control study, there was a significant trend in decreasing risk with the number of

Table 5.12 The association between single nucleotide polymorphisms and PD

Gene	SNPs	Genotype or model	Adjusted odds ratio	95% confidence interval or *P* value
LARK2 Gly2385Arg [21]	rs34778348	GA vs. GG	2.06	1.15 to 3.69
MAOB [22]	rs1799836	AG vs. AA	0.61	0.37 to 0.99
		Additive model (G)	Not shown	($p = 0.016$)
		AA vs. AG + GG	1.70	1.12 to 2.58
COMT [22]	rs4680	Additive model (A)	Not shown	$p = 0.044$
SNCA [24]	rs356220	CC + CT vs. TT	1.42	1.002 to 2.02
	rs2736990	Additive model (G)	1.30	1.002 to 1.68
UCHL1 S18Y [25]		CC vs. CA + AA	1.57	1.06 to 2.31
PARK16 [28]	rs823128	AG vs. AA	0.64	0.42 to 0.97
		Additive model (G)	0.64	0.44 to 0.93
		AA vs. AG + GG	0.62	0.41 to 0.93
	rs947211	GG vs. AA	3.06	1.83 to 5.12
		Additive model (G)	1.76	1.36 to 2.28
		AA vs. AG+ GG	1.99	1.29 to 3.07
	rs823156	Additive model (G)	0.68	0.48 to 0.96
		AA vs. AG + GG	0.67	0.46 to 0.98
VDR [29]	rs2228570	Additive model (A)	0.77	0.60 to 0.997

the G alleles of *MAOB* rs1799836 ($p = 0.016$) [22]. Catechol-O-methyltransferase (COMT) is an enzyme associated with metabolism of dopamine. There was a significant trend in increasing risk with the number of the A alleles of COMT rs4680 ($p = 0.044$) [22].

Previous studies showed that the *LARK2* Gly2385Arg variant is a risk factor for PD. In the present case-control study, compared with the GG genotype, the GA genotype had a significantly increased risk of PD in the multivariate model [21]. Furthermore, compared with subjects with the GG genotype, those with the GA genotype who had never smoked had a 5.8-fold increased risk of PD; however, the multiplicative interaction between the SNP and smoking was not statistically significant. With respect to the additive interaction, the estimated attributable proportion due to interaction (AP), but not relative excess risk due to interaction (RERI) or the synergy index (S), was statistically significant.

The α-synuclein protein (140 amino acid) is encoded by the *SNCA* gene. α-Synuclein protein is the major fibrillary component of Lewy neurites, suggesting the association with PD. *SNCA* SNPs rs356220 and 2736990, but not rs356229, rs356219, or rs7684318, were significantly associated with the risk of PD [24]. The significant additive interactions were observed between SNPs rs356219 and rs356220 and smoking with respect to PD, although the multiplicative interactions were not significant.

Ubiquitin carboxy-terminal hydrolase L1 (UCHL1) activity has been shown to be required for normal synaptic function. Compared with subjects with the CC or CA genotype of *UCHL S18Y* SNP, those with the AA genotype had a significantly increased risk PD [25].

PARK16 was identified as a new PD susceptibility locus in a genome-wide association study in the Japanese. *PARK16* SNPs rs823128, rs947211, and rs823156, but not rs16856139 or rs11240572, were significantly associated with the risk of PD (Table 5.12) [28]. Compared with subjects with the AA genotype of SNP rs823128 who had ever smoked, those with the AG or GG genotype who had never smoked had a 3.3-fold increased risk of sporadic PD: the additive interaction between SNP rs823128 and smoking affecting sporadic PD was significant because the 95% CIs of the RERI and AP values were >0, while the multiplicative interaction was not significant.

Previous studies showed that PD patients had lower mean levels of 25-hydroxyvitamin D than healthy controls. Because the biological actions of the active form of vitamin D are mediated by the nuclear vitamin D receptor (VDR), SNPs in the VDR gene may have roles in the development of PD. *VDR* SNPs rs2228570, but not rs731236, rs7975232, or rs1544410, was significantly associated with the risk of PD [29].

In the study on APOE polymorphisms, compared with the APOE ε3/ε3 genotype, the 2/ε4 genotype was associated with an increased risk of PD (adjusted OR = 9.50, 95% CI: 1.12 to 80.6) [23]. The presence of the ε3 allele was associated with a decreased risk of PD: adjusted OR in additive model = 0.08, 95% CI; 0.01 to 0.62).

No association was observed between *GST* [20], *BST1* [26], or *MDR1* [27] and the risk of PD.

5.4 Discussion

The Fukuoka Kinki Parkinson's Disease Study had methodological strengths. All PD patients were diagnosed by a neurologist according to established criteria, therefore, there is little reason to suspect that there was a serious misdiagnosis of PD. The response rate among cases was relatively high (84%). We took into consideration comprehensive information on potential confounders.

Important weaknesses of the present study should be considered. Information on lifestyle and environmental factors such as smoking habits, diet, and occupation was based on self-reports. Consequently, the possibility of inaccurate exposure data and resulting misclassification bias should be considered when interpreting our findings.

Another problem with retrospective case-control studies is recall bias. However, risk factors for PD are poorly characterized; therefore, study subjects have few systematic preconceived ideas regarding their disease etiology. We used the DHQ which was designed to assess dietary intake for 1 month prior to completing the questionnaire. Current rather than past dietary habits were assessed because retrospective estimation of past dietary consumption is generally difficult and the utility of our DHQ for dietary intake in the past is unknown. Therefore, our case-control study was inevitably based on the assumption that the patterns of relative food intake of cases and control subjects remained fairly stable over time. Pre-symptomatic and/or post-symptomatic PD such as their food preferences in the preclinical stage and food choices affected by some of the non-motor symptoms could influence dietary habits in some cases which would lead to misclassification of their true long-term dietary exposure. The study size was rather small for a valid genetic association study. The lack of significant relationships between some SNPs which we examined and the risk of PD might be attributable to insufficient statistical power.

In order to establish evidence on preventive and risk factors for PD in Japanese, further case-control studies with a larger number of subjects and also by functional studies are needed.

References

1. Nussbaum RL, Ellis CE. Alzheimer's disease and Parkinson's disease. N Engl J Med. 2003;348:1356–64.
2. Li X, Li W, Liu G, Shen X, Tang Y. Association between cigarette smoking and Parkinson's disease: a meta-analysis. Arch Gerontol Geriatr. 2015;61:510–6.
3. Tanaka K, Miyake Y, Fukushima W, Sasaki S, Kiyohara C, Tsuboi Y, Yamada T, Oeda T, Miki T, Kawamura N, Sakae N, Fukuyama H, Hirota Y, Nagai M, Fukuoka Kinki Parkinson's disease Study Group. Active and passive smoking and risk of Parkinson's disease. Acta Neurol Scand. 2010;122:377–82.
4. Hughes AJ, Daniel SE, Kilford L, Lees AJ. Accuracy of clinical diagnosis of idiopathic Parkinson's disease: a clinico-pathological study of 100 cases. J Neurol Neurosurg Psychiatry. 1992;55:181–4.
5. Sasaki S, Yanagibori R, Amano K. Self-administered diet history questionnaire developed for health education: a relative validation of the test-version by comparison with 3-day diet record in women. J Epidemiol. 1998;8:203–15.
6. Sasaki S, Ushio F, Amano K, et al. Serum biomarker-based validation of a self-administered diet history questionnaire for Japanese subjects. J Nutr Sci Vitaminol. 2000;46:285–96.
7. Science and Technology Agency. Standard tables of food composition in Japan, 5th revised and enlarged ed. Tokyo, Japan: printing Bureau of the Ministry of Finance, 2005 (in Japanese).
8. Science and Technology Agency. Standard Tables of Food Composition in Japan, Fatty Acid Section, 5th revised and enlarged ed. Tokyo, Japan: Printing Bureau of the Ministry of Finance, 2005 (in Japanese).
9. Willett W, Stampfer MJ. Total energy intake: implications for epidemiologic analyses. Am J Epidemiol. 1986;124:17–27.
10. Tanaka K, Miyake Y, Fukushima W, Sasaki S, Kiyohara C, Tsuboi Y, Yamada T, Oeda T, Miki T, Kawamura N, Sakae N, Fukuyama H, Hirota Y, Nagai M, Fukuoka Kinki Parkinson's Disease Study Group. Occupational risk factors for Parkinson's disease: a case-control study in Japan. BMC Neurol. 2011;11:83.

11. Miyake Y, Tanaka K, Fukushima W, Sasaki S, Kiyohara C, Tsuboi Y, Yamada T, Oeda T, Miki T, Kawamura N, Sakae N, Fukuyama H, Hirota Y, Nagai M, Fukuoka Kinki Parkinson's Disease Study Group. Case-control study of risk of Parkinson's disease in relation to hypertension, hypercholesterolemia, and diabetes in Japan. J Neurol Sci. 2010;293:82–6.
12. Fukushima W, Miyake Y, Tanaka K, Sasaki S, Kiyohara C, Tsuboi Y, Yamada T, Oeda T, Miki T, Kawamura N, Sakae N, Fukuyama H, Hirota Y, Nagai M, Fukuoka Kinki Parkinson's Disease Study Group. Alcohol drinking and risk of Parkinson's disease: a case-control study in Japan. BMC Neurol. 2010;10:111.
13. Tanaka K, Miyake Y, Fukushima W, Sasaki S, Kiyohara C, Tsuboi Y, Yamada T, Oeda T, Miki T, Kawamura N, Sakae N, Fukuyama H, Hirota Y, Nagai M, Fukuoka Kinki Parkinson's Disease Study Group. Intake of Japanese and Chinese teas reduces risk of Parkinson's disease. Parkinsonism Relat Disord. 2011;17:446–50.
14. Miyake Y, Fukushima W, Tanaka K, Sasaki S, Kiyohara C, Tsuboi Y, Yamada T, Oeda T, Miki T, Kawamura N, Sakae N, Fukuyama H, Hirota Y, Nagai M, Fukuoka Kinki Parkinson's Disease Study Group. Dietary intake of antioxidant vitamins and risk of Parkinson's disease: a case-control study in Japan. Eur J Neurol. 2011;18:106–13.
15. Miyake Y, Tanaka K, Fukushima W, Sasaki S, Kiyohara C, Tsuboi Y, Yamada T, Oeda T, Miki T, Kawamura N, Sakae N, Fukuyama H, Hirota Y, Nagai M, Fukuoka Kinki Parkinson's Disease Study Group. Lack of association of dairy food, calcium, and vitamin D intake with the risk of Parkinson's disease: a case-control study in Japan. Parkinsonism Relat Disord. 2011;17:112–6.
16. Miyake Y, Tanaka K, Fukushima W, Sasaki S, Kiyohara C, Tsuboi Y, Yamada T, Oeda T, Miki T, Kawamura N, Sakae N, Fukuyama H, Hirota Y, Nagai M, Fukuoka Kinki Parkinson's Disease Study Group. Dietary intake of metals and risk of Parkinson's disease: a case-control study in Japan. J Neurol Sci. 2011;306:98–102.
17. Miyake Y, Sasaki S, Tanaka K, Fukushima W, Kiyohara C, Tsuboi Y, Yamada T, Oeda T, Miki T, Kawamura N, Sakae N, Fukuyama H, Hirota Y, Nagai M, Fukuoka Kinki Parkinson's Disease Study Group. Dietary fat intake and risk of Parkinson's disease: a case-control study in Japan. J Neurol Sci. 2010;288:117–22.
18. Murakami K, Miyake Y, Sasaki S, Tanaka K, Fukushima W, Kiyohara C, Tsuboi Y, Yamada T, Oeda T, Miki T, Kawamura N, Sakae N, Fukuyama H, Hirota Y, Nagai M, Fukuoka Kinki Parkinson's Disease Study Group. Dietary glycemic index is inversely associated with the risk of Parkinson's disease: a case-control study in Japan. Nutrition. 2010;26:515–21.
19. Okubo H, Miyake Y, Sasaki S, Murakami K, Tanaka K, Fukushima W, Kiyohara C, Tsuboi Y, Yamada T, Oeda T, Shimada H, Kawamura N, Sakae N, Fukuyama H, Hirota Y, Nagai M, Fukuoka Kinki Parkinson's Disease Study Group. Dietary patterns and risk of Parkinson's disease: a case-control study in Japan. Eur J Neurol. 2012;19:681–8.
20. Kiyohara C, Miyake Y, Koyanagi M, Fujimoto T, Shirasawa S, Tanaka K, Fukushima W, Sasaki S, Tsuboi Y, Yamada T, Oeda T, Miki T, Kawamura N, Sakae N, Fukuyama H, Hirota Y, Nagai M, Fukuoka Kinki Parkinson's Disease Study Group. *GST* polymorphisms, interaction with smoking and pesticide use, and risk for Parkinson's disease in a Japanese population. Parkinsonism Relat Disord. 2010;16:447–52.
21. Miyake Y, Tsuboi Y, Koyanagi M, Fujimoto T, Shirasawa S, Kiyohara C, Tanaka K, Fukushima W, Sasaki S, Yamada T, Oeda T, Miki T, Kawamura N, Sakae N, Fukuyama H, Hirota Y, Nagai M, Fukuoka Kinki Parkinson's Disease Study Group. *LRRK2* Gly2385Arg polymorphism, cigarette smoking, and risk of sporadic Parkinson's disease: a case-control study in Japan. J Neurol Sci. 2010;297:15–8.
22. Kiyohara C, Miyake Y, Koyanagi M, Fujimoto T, Shirasawa S, Tanaka K, Fukushima W, Sasaki S, Tsuboi Y, Yamada T, Oeda T, Shimada H, Kawamura N, Sakae N, Fukuyama H, Hirota Y, Nagai M, Fukuoka Kinki Parkinson's Disease Study Group. Genetic polymorphisms involved in dopaminergic neurotransmission and risk for Parkinson's disease in a Japanese population. BMC Neurol. 2011;11:89.
23. Kiyohara C, Miyake Y, Koyanagi M, Fujimoto T, Shirasawa S, Tanaka K, Fukushima W, Sasaki S, Tsuboi Y, Yamada T, Oeda T, Miki T, Kawamura N, Sakae N, Fukuyama H, Hirota

Y, Nagai M, Fukuoka Kinki Parkinson's Disease Study Group. *APOE* and *CYP2E1* polymorphisms, alcohol consumption, and Parkinson's disease in a Japanese population. J Neural Transm. 2011;118:1335–44.
24. Miyake Y, Tanaka K, Fukushima W, Kiyohara C, Sasaki S, Tsuboi Y, Yamada T, Oeda T, Shimada H, Kawamura N, Sakae N, Fukuyama H, Hirota Y, Nagai M, Fukuoka Kinki Parkinson's Disease Study Group. *SNCA* polymorphisms, smoking, and sporadic Parkinson's disease in Japanese. Parkinsonism Relat Disord. 2012;18:557–61.
25. Miyake Y, Tanaka K, Fukushima W, Kiyohara C, Sasaki S, Tsuboi Y, Yamada T, Oeda T, Shimada H, Kawamura N, Sakae N, Fukuyama H, Hirota Y, Nagai M, Fukuoka Kinki Parkinson's Disease Study Group. *UCHL1* S18Y variant is a risk factor for Parkinson's disease in Japan. BMC Neurol. 2012;12:62.
26. Miyake Y, Tanaka K, Fukushima W, Kiyohara C, Sasaki S, Tsuboi Y, Yamada T, Oeda T, Shimada H, Kawamura N, Sakae N, Fukuyama H, Hirota Y, Nagai M, Fukuoka Kinki Parkinson's Disease Study Group. Lack of association between *BST1* polymorphisms and sporadic Parkinson's disease in a Japanese population. J Neurol Sci. 2012;323:162–6.
27. Kiyohara C, Miyake Y, Koyanagi M, Fujimoto T, Shirasawa S, Tanaka K, Fukushima W, Sasaki S, Tsuboi Y, Yamada T, Oeda T, Shimada H, Kawamura N, Sakae N, Fukuyama H, Hirota Y, Nagai M, Fukuoka Kinki Parkinson's Disease Study Group. *MDR1* C3435T polymorphism and interaction with environmental factors in risk of Parkinson's disease: a case-control study in Japan. Drug Metab Pharmacokinet. 2013;28:138–43.
28. Miyake Y, Tanaka K, Fukushima W, Kiyohara C, Sasaki S, Tsuboi Y, Oeda T, Shimada H, Kawamura N, Sakae N, Fukuyama H, Hirota Y, Nagai M, Nakamura Y, Fukuoka Kinki Parkinson's Disease Study Group. *PARK16* polymorphisms, interaction with smoking, and sporadic Parkinson's disease in Japan. J Neurol Sci. 2016;362:47–52.
29. Tanaka K, Miyake Y, Fukushima W, Kiyohara C, Sasaki S, Tsuboi Y, Oeda T, Shimada H, Kawamura N, Sakae N, Fukuyama H, Hirota Y, Nagai M, Nakamura Y, Fukuoka Kinki Parkinson's Disease Study Group. Vitamin D receptor gene polymorphisms, smoking, and risk of sporadic Parkinson's disease in Japan. Neurosci Lett. 2017;643:97–102.

Chapter 6
Descriptive and Analytic Epidemiology of Idiopathic Normal Pressure Hydrocephalus (iNPH) in Japan

Nagato Kuriyama, Masakazu Miyajima, Madoka Nakajima, Takeo Kato, Michiko Kurosawa, Wakaba Fukushima, Takahiko Tokuda, Yoshiyuki Watanabe, Etsuko Ozaki, Teruhide Koyama, Daisuke Matsui, Isao Watanabe, and Hajime Arai

Abstract The two pillars of descriptive and analytic epidemiological studies on intractable diseases are clarification of the number of patients showing symptoms and basic clinical features. This report introduces the importance of descriptive and analytic epidemiology of intractable diseases with regard to the significance, meth-

N. Kuriyama (✉)
Department of Epidemiology for Community Health and Medicine, Kyoto Prefectural University of Medicine, Kyoto, Japan

Department of Neurology, Kyoto Prefectural University of Medicine, Kamigyo-ku, Kyoto, Japan
e-mail: nkuriyam@koto.kpu-m.ac.jp

M. Miyajima · M. Nakajima · H. Arai
Department of Neurosurgery, Juntendo University Graduate School of Medicine, Tokyo, Japan

T. Kato
Faculty of Medicine, Department of Neurology, Hematology, Metabolism, Endocrinology and Diabetology, Yamagata University, Yamagata, Japan

M. Kurosawa
Department of Epidemiology and Environmental Health, Juntendo University Graduate School of Medicine, Tokyo, Japan

W. Fukushima
Department of Public Health, Osaka City University Faculty of Medicine, Osaka, Japan

T. Tokuda
Department of Neurology, Kyoto Prefectural University of Medicine, Kamigyo-ku, Kyoto, Japan

Y. Watanabe · E. Ozaki · T. Koyama · D. Matsui · I. Watanabe
Department of Epidemiology for Community Health and Medicine, Kyoto Prefectural University of Medicine, Kyoto, Japan

M. Washio, G. Kobashi (eds.), *Epidemiological Studies of Specified Rare and Intractable Disease*, Current Topics in Environmental Health and Preventive Medicine, https://doi.org/10.1007/978-981-13-1096-6_6

odology, and points of attention through a nationwide survey of idiopathic normal pressure hydrocephalus (iNPH) that we experienced including specific survey methods, with introduction of reports from Japan and other countries.

iNPH manifests three features: gait disturbance, cognitive impairment, and urinary incontinence. The cerebrospinal fluid pressure is within the normal range although ventricular enlargement occurs, and symptoms can be improved by cerebrospinal fluid shunt treatment. It is more likely to develop in the elderly (60 years old or older), attracting attention as a geriatric disease of unknown cause with increasing number of patients. After the treatment guidelines were established, new epidemiological information has been accumulating in Japan. This nationwide hospital-based epidemiologic survey was performed based on patient's background and clarified the presence of 13,000 patients treated for iNPH per year in Japan. In addition, comorbidities of iNPH included hypertension, diabetes, Alzheimer disease, and orthopedic diseases, and gender-specific characteristics were noted. Long-term treatment effect can be obtained by appropriate diagnosis and proper cerebrospinal fluid shunt operation. Utilization of the data collected by previous studies on iNPH reported in Japan and other countries including this nationwide survey is expected to elucidate the fundamental mechanism related to the cause and pathology of iNPH as a treatable disease of the elderly.

Keywords Nationwide hospital-based epidemiologic survey · Idiopathic normal pressure hydrocephalus · Prevalence · Incidence · Comorbidity

6.1 Introduction

Descriptive and analytic epidemiology of intractable diseases has been attracting attention in the field of social medicine. The basic countermeasures against intractable diseases are strengthening of diagnosis and treatment of each intractable disease, for which accurate summation of medical information, such as the total number of patients, morbidity, prevalence, and characteristic of age distribution in each disease, and preparation of information collected by descriptive and analytic epidemiological surveys to be utilized in actual medical practice are important. Utilizing the clinical survey registration forms of individuals or administrative-level hospital documents and medical prescription data of each disease, nationwide epidemiological surveys were performed mainly by the health and medical administrations in each country and promoted development of various descriptive and analytic epidemiological methods for intractable diseases.

The pillars of descriptive and analytic epidemiological studies on intractable diseases are clarification of the number of patients and basic clinical features. Specifically, various types of research and studies are performed to discover the disease early, identify preventive factors, and evaluate the outcomes of advanced treatments by analyzing the frequency of each intractable disease (including the total number of patients, morbidity, and prevalence), characteristics of the age distribution, and clinical background, for which the role of epidemiology liaison exerts in survey studies on intractable diseases are as important as that of clinical specialists actually registering individual patients in routine medical practice.

In this report, the significance, methodology, and points of attention of survey studies are introduced based on a hospital-based nationwide survey of an intractable disease, idiopathic normal pressure hydrocephalus (iNPH), that we experienced. In addition, the importance of descriptive and analytic epidemiology and the role of epidemiology liaison exerts are discussed while introducing reports on iNPH from Japan and other countries.

6.2 Historical Background of Idiopathic Normal Pressure Hydrocephalus

In Japan entering the aged society, idiopathic normal pressure hydrocephalus (iNPH) has recently been attracting attention as a geriatric disease with an increase in the incidence in the elderly (60 years old or older), although the cause is still unclear, and how to perform early medical and nursing care interventions for a geriatric disease, iNPH, in upcoming super-aging society is an important theme of geriatric medicine.

Idiopathic normal pressure hydrocephalus (iNPH) causes three features: gait disturbance, cognitive impairment, and urinary incontinence. The cerebrospinal fluid pressure is within the normal range although ventricular enlargement occurs, and symptoms can be improved by cerebrospinal fluid shunt operation. Hakim and Adams initially proposed it as an independent single disease concept in 1965 [1, 2]. iNPH is an important geriatric disease expected to increase patients as a treatable cognitive impairment in the aging society. Since all of the above symptoms negatively influence ADL, accurate early discovery, diagnosis, and treatment are necessary, and its clinical background and pathology have been attracting attention.

Although iNPH is a disease specific to the elderly, as shown by its name "idiopathic," no preceding diseases develop, such as subarachnoid hemorrhage and meningitis, and it chronically progresses slowly due to impaired absorption of cerebrospinal fluid [3, 4]. This disease is similar to normal aging and other dementia (such as Alzheimer disease and Binswanger's disease) or may be complicated by these depending on cases, and causes nonspecific symptoms frequently observed in the elderly, being likely to be overlooked. However, it is possible to improve symptoms by appropriate cerebrospinal fluid shunt operation in elderly patients (60 years old or older), being known as a treatable disease, i.e., the treatment method was discovered before elucidation of the cause [3–5]. The fundamental cause and pathology have not yet been elucidated as shown by its name, "idiopathic," while an effective treatment method, shunt operation, was discovered beforehand, showing uniqueness and characteristics of this disease. Therefore, it has not been completely elucidated what step of the process of cerebrospinal fluid absorption is impaired in iNPH or whether ventricular enlargement results from this. However, the pathology and clinical characteristics of iNPH suggest the presence of impaired cerebrospinal fluid absorption in the brain parenchyma or near the subarachnoid space, and the disease is considered an important research subject concerning cerebrospinal fluid circulation in basic medicine in the future. Fortunately, the clinical guidelines for iNPH have been formulated and a nationwide epidemiological survey has been performed with support by the Ministry of Health, Labour and Welfare as a core disease under the Research on Measures for Intractable Diseases Project in Japan, and the disease has become widely known as an intractable disease with a curable treatment method, with which pioneering reports leading to further elucidation of the pathology are needed. At the same time, further progression of clinical-epidemiological, pathological, and physiological studies is expected.

Although the revised edition of the iNPH-related treatment guidelines [6–8] was formulated and a certain number of hospital-based or population-based studies have been reported (Table 6.1), from a descriptive and analytic epidemiological point of view, no accurate national-level epidemiological survey or study on iNPH has been sufficiently performed. No nationwide clinical epidemiology of iNPH, such as the total number of patients, morbidity, prevalence, clinical characteristics, and actual clinical state, has been reported in any country, not limited to Japan. Accordingly, accurate epidemiological information of iNPH has been needed, requiring a national-level epidemiological survey. In 2013, conditions for an epidemiological survey of iNPH, such as research staff and funding, became ready and we performed the initial national-level hospital-based nationwide epidemiological survey of iNPH mainly led by epidemiology liaison exerts. The annual number of patients treated, estimated prevalence, clinical background, and risk factors were clarified, and a report written in English was published by the Ministry of Health, Labour and Welfare Research Group [9].

6.3 History of Guideline Preparation for Idiopathic Normal Pressure Hydrocephalus and Accompanying Clinical Studies

Generally, to perform an epidemiological survey/study on intractable disease, formulation of medical care measures and guidelines capable of providing accurate and appropriate information are required as prerequisites. Since recognition of iNPH largely varied among regions, facilities, and physicians, guidelines for treatment of this disease were published in 2004, aiming at standardization of diagnosis and treatment of iNPH [10]. Subsequently, the second revised edition of the iNPH-related treatment guidelines [7] was published in 2011 to promote the spread and understanding of the characteristics, importance, and aiming at latest knowledge on this disease. The first author (N.K.) and coauthors (M.M., M.N., T.T., T.K., and H.A.) participated in the formulation. The US iNPH treatment guidelines were also published in the same period [6, 8], but attention should be paid to that cases with

Table 6.1 Recent major reported epidemiological survey of iNPH in the literature

Author-year	Country	Subjects of investigation	Epidemiological data
Hospital-based study			
Vanneste et al. 1992	Netherlands	166 shunt operation cases with iNPH among 2500,000 residents in multiple hospital-based nationwide collaborative survey in Netherlands	Incidence rate of shunt-responsive iNPH: 2.2/million/year
Tisell et al. 2005	Sweden	891 patients who underwent surgery for hydrocephalus in one the six university hospitals in Sweden during 1996–1998	Incidence of iNPH surgery: 1.6/100.000/year (47% of 3.4/100.000/year)
Brean et al. 2009	Norway	4,644,761 inhabitants of Norway in 2006.	Incidence of iNPH: 1.09/100,000/year (> 65 years 30.2/100,000/year)
Klassen et al. 2011	USA	124,277 inhabitants in a community of Minnesota, USA	Incidence of clinically suspected iNPH:1.19/100,000/year
Muangpaisan et al. 2012	Thailand	233 dementia patients of an outpatient geriatric clinic in a hospital	Prevalence rate of iNPH:0.9%
Kuriyama et al. 2017	Japan	The residents who had a medical diagnosis as iNPH by hospital-based nationwide survey in Japan	Crude prevalence of iNPH in the whole Japanese population: 10.2/100,000/year estimated prevalence in over 70-year-olds of iNPH: 58/100,000/year
Population-based study			
Brean et al. 2008	Norway	220,000 inhabitants who had a medical examination by the health-promotive activity in a city.	Prevalence and incidence of probable iNPH: 21.9 and 5.5 /100,000/year
Hiraoka et al. 2008	Japan (Miyagi prefecture)	170 randomly selected local residents >65-year-olds out of 2516 elderly inhabitants of the town Tajiri	Prevalence rate of MRI-supported possible iNPH:2.9% patients ≥65 years
Tanaka et al. 2009	Japan (Miyagi prefecture)	567 local residents who were randomly selected from the 1654 local inhabitants ≥65 years old	Prevalence rate of MRI-supported possible iNPH: 1.4%≥ of 65 years
Iseki et al. 2009	Japan (Yamagata prefecture)	790 local residents (69.2%) who were 61 years old and all 70–72-year-olds	Prevalence rate of MRI-supported possible iNPH:0.5%
Iseki et al. 2014	Japan (Yamagata prefecture)	271 local inhabitants who were all 70-year-olds	Incidence of possible iNPH: 1.2/100(120/100,000) prevalence rate of possible iNPH:0.37%

(continued)

Table 6.1 (continued)

Author-year	Country	Subjects of investigation	Epidemiological data
Jaraj et al. 2014	Sweden	1238 residents >70 years old with brain CT and neuropsychological examination.	Prevalence rate of probable iNPH: 0.2% in 70–79-year-olds, 5.9% in >80-year-olds.
Nakashita et al. 2016	Japan (Tottori prefecture)	607 local residents ≥65 years old with brain MRI and cognitive examinations	Prevalence rate of possible iNPH:2.8%
Health insurance-database based study			
Lemcke et al. 2016	Germany	7.5 million insurants of nationwide health insurance claim data	Incidence of iNPH: 1.36/100,000/year prevalence rate of iNPH:0.01%

delayed onset of congenital hydrocephalus symptoms may be included in the US iNPH guidelines because the onset age of iNPH symptoms is described as 40 years old or older [6, 8]. Actually, in studies investigating a large number of iNPH patients, the mean age was about 75 years old and the number of patients in their 40s was considered small [11, 12].

iNPH is now known worldwide and routine medical practice, diagnosis, examination, and treatment are performed based on standardized diagnostic criteria. Upon publication of the guidelines [6–8], a much greater understanding of the pathology and treatment of this disease has developed. In this context, the iNPH guidelines play a specific role in spreading clinical information of iNPH. The iNPH guidelines [7] specify three diagnosis levels (possible, probable, and definite) and the optimum medical care for each level. Application of cerebrospinal fluid shunt operation rapidly increased as awareness of iNPH markedly increased, and basic and clinical studies on iNPH have markedly progressed.

In Japan, iNPH was selected for Research on Measures for Intractable Diseases Project under the initiative by the Ministry of Health, Labour and Welfare, and a Research Group has been organized. In the process of guideline formulation described above, the necessity of transmitting high evidence-level research results became understood. A multicenter prospective cohort study: Study of Idiopathic Normal Pressure Hydrocephalus on Neurological Improvement (SINPHONI), was conducted mainly by this iNPH Research Group in Japan [13]. As a result of this study, application of cerebrospinal fluid shunt operation was approved regardless of the results of CSF exclusion test (cerebrospinal tap test) for cases clinically suspected with iNPH showing the features of disproportionately enlarged subarachnoid-space hydrocephalus (DESH) specified by the diagnostic criteria on brain MRI, i.e., ventricular enlargement with narrowing of the subarachnoid space in the high-convexity area. Therefore, imaging diagnosis is important for treatment of iNPH, and morphological evaluation using brain CT and MRI became essential to diagnose iNPH. As a result of the world's initial randomized controlled study, SINPHONI-2 [14] have been reported from Japan, the efficacy of cerebrospinal fluid shunt operation for iNPH was ensured.

While clinical information concerning iNPH is being accumulated, for example, which of the three features described above is frequently encountered at clinical practice sites depends on the department that patients visit first, for example, many patients visit the orthopedic department for gait disturbance. However, very few descriptive epidemiological studies accurately reflected the overall actual state of routine medical practice. Thus, international comparison of data concerning iNPH has not been performed with regard to the epidemiology and treatment effect. Many other unsolved tasks remain for iNPH with regard to the cause of disease, diagnosis, and treatment method. Selection of cerebrospinal fluid biomarkers useful to diagnose and differentiate iNPH, follow-up survey of asymptomatic iNPH, establishment of severity classification applicable for evaluation of treatment, and medical economic investigation are planned, and interesting reports in these directions may come out in the future.

6.4 Treatment of Idiopathic Normal Pressure Hydrocephalus

The main pathology of iNPH is impairment of cerebrospinal fluid circulation, and it has been reported that the cerebrospinal fluid turn-over rate decreases to 1/4 of that in healthy individuals [15]. Accordingly, the objective of iNPH treatment is correction of impaired cerebrospinal fluid circulation, and the main body of treatment is cerebrospinal fluid shunt operation [6–8]. Previously, ventriculo-peritoneal shunt (VP shunt) was performed as the first-line treatment in many cases. However, it had a risk of damaging the brain because a tube is inserted into the brain. Since a study demonstrating the efficacy of lumbo-peritoneal shunt (LP shunt) not damaging the brain was reported in 2015 [14], LP shunt has been frequently applied instead of VP shunt, becoming the first-choice. This clinical study [14] investigated the usefulness of lumbar subarachnoid peritoneal shunt of cerebrospinal fluid (LP shunt operation). It was an investigator-initiated multicenter clinical study and designated as Study of Idiopathic Normal Pressure Hydrocephalus on Neurological Improvement-2 (SINPHONI-2) and performed at 20 medical institutions in Japan. Specifically, after registration of 93 iNPH patients, they were randomly divided into two groups: a group undergoing L-P shunt (early group comprised of 49 patients) and a group waiting for undergoing L-P shunt for 3 months with exercise along a program (waiting group comprised of 44 patients). Changes in the symptoms after 3 months compared with those at the time of registration were compared between the early and waiting groups, and the usefulness of L-P shunt operation, which does not damage the brain, was clarified initially in the world. When the results of this clinical study are clearly presented in the guidelines, L-P shunt may become the first-recommendation level. However, it is still not described in the treatment guidelines. At present, the shunt method to be selected as the first-choice for individual cases is decided based on the physical condition of the patient and operator's experience in consideration of the age, complications, and requests from patients [16, 17].

6.5 Nationwide Epidemiological Survey of Idiopathic Normal Pressure Hydrocephalus

Many iNPH patients live an inactive life because gait disturbance and cognitive impairment accompanied by loss of motivation develop at a high frequency [18]. These patients are suspected as having iNPH and visit the hospital for close examination, initially undergoing imaging of the head and cognitive function and gait tests. However, no national-level survey of epidemiological and clinical backgrounds useful for both patients and medical personnel has been previously reported. Moreover, confirmation of improvement of clinical symptoms by painful invasive examination, such as CSF removal test, is necessary to definitely diagnose the disease, and this is not easy for general internists to perform and likely to be overlooked. Accordingly, previously reported hospital-based surveys were limited to hospitals where patients gathered, being the main trend (Table 6.1), i.e., these studies have limitations that it was performed in limited hospitals and thus limited the number of patients definitely diagnosed with iNPH. There may have been many patients who did not visit the surveyed hospitals being not registered. Therefore, it is possible that the number of treated patients was far greater than previously expected.

After the guidelines were formulated, population-based surveys have recently been performed as shown in Table 6.1, increasing epidemiological information of iNPH, but consideration of the regional characteristics is necessary for all these surveys and the epidemiological description remains vague throughout the world.

Based on the situation that no national-level nationwide survey of iNPH has been performed, a nationwide epidemiological survey centering the total annual number of iNPH patients was performed in 2013 mainly by the iNPH Research Group supported by the Ministry of Health, Labour and Welfare [9], and the epidemiological features, clinical characteristics, background factors, and risk factors of iNPH were clarified by the hospital-based nationwide survey. The methods and the essence of the results are introduced below.

6.5.1 Materials and Methods

The nationwide epidemiological survey consisted of two stages: the primary survey aiming at summation of the total number of patients and the secondary survey aiming at collecting clinical information. The survey was carried out mainly by the Clinical Research Group and epidemiology liaison experts in cooperation with nationwide clinical hospitals. The method is specifically described below.

6.5.1.1 Methods for Hospital-Based Nationwide Survey

This survey consisted of two epidemiological surveys. As a primary survey, the total number of patients who were diagnosed with NPH and received medical care in 2012 (the estimated number of cases that meet the diagnostic criteria of iNPH) and the number of patients who received shunt operation (the estimated numbers of cases performed shunt operation) were surveyed using postal mail. In the subsequent secondary survey, attending physicians reported the concrete clinical information of the registered patients in the primary survey by filling the secondary survey form aiming at clarifying the clinical characteristics of this disease and sent it by postal mail.

6.5.1.2 Diagnostic Criteria

For the diagnostic criteria of iNPH used in this survey, '2011 revised edition of the Guidelines for management of idiopathic normal pressure hydrocephalus' [7] was used. In addition, based on the management guidelines, the numbers of patients classified into the three diagnostic levels: possible, probable, and definite, and outlines were also surveyed. Briefly, the main point of each diagnostic level is as follows: When the disease onsets at 60 years old or older with symptoms of one or more of gait disturbance, cognitive impairment, and urinary incontinence with no preceding disease, and ventricular enlargement is noted with normal cerebrospinal fluid pressure, the case is possible iNPH. When gait disturbance and disproportionately enlarged subarachnoid space hydrocephalus (DESH) on imaging are additionally present, or reactivity was noted on the cerebrospinal fluid exclusion test, the case is probable iNPH. Cerebrospinal fluid shunt operation is applied to treat probable iNPH, and when the clinical symptoms improved, the case is definite iNPH [7].

6.5.1.3 Target Departments and Medical Institutions of the Survey

Referring to previous nationwide surveys of other diseases, we performed the primary and secondary surveys to select the target departments, medical institutions, and special stratified hospitals following the method standardized by the Research Committee on Epidemiology of Intractable Diseases in Japan [19, 20].

The targets of the survey were selected by the number of beds using the random sampling method. For the department, neurosurgery, neurology, neuropsychiatry, and internal medicine were selected. The number of patients by the department in 2012 was asked in the primary survey, then, description of the detailed patient information was requested in the secondary survey. The number of patients treated for iNPH was estimated based on the primary survey, and the characteristics of the clinical epidemiology were investigated in the secondary survey. The target department was specified to neurosurgery, neurology, neuropsychiatry, and internal medicine, and the primary survey was conducted in January 2013.

Specifically, the medical institution list was prepared based on the electronic database of Japanese Byoin-Yohran and list of university medical training institutions to train clinicians, and the institutions were selected for each department by the number of beds employing the stratified random sampling method. The lists are widely available in electronic database form and list all the hospitals from north to south in Japan. The percentages in the sampling method were determined corresponding to the number of beds in hospitals following the procedure below: Stratification was conducted according to the number of hospital beds. Sampling fractions were as follows: general hospitals with 99 or fewer beds (5%); 100 to 199 beds (10%); 200 to 299 beds (20%); 300 to 399 beds (40%); 400 to 499 beds (80%); 500 or more beds (100%); and university Hospitals (100%). For example, regarding a stratum of general hospitals with 200 to 299 beds, we randomly selected one department and then selected the next one by a five-department interval, yielding 20% of the sampling fraction. As special stratified hospitals for iNPH, 75 departments that treated a large number of patients with idiopathic NPH were included by 100% sampling fractions [9]. Clinics with 19 or fewer beds were widely registered as the target in the present nationwide epidemiological survey conducted by us, which was a new attempt.

6.5.1.4 Survey Items of the Survey Form and Analysis

Responses to the second questionnaire in the secondary survey on the detailed patient information were requested to the facilities and departments which responded that iNPH patients were present in the primary survey. The following items were asked in the primary survey: The presence or absence of patients meeting the diagnostic criteria in 2012 in each department, estimated number of iNPH patients seeking medical care, and estimated number of patients treated with shunt operation. Based on the above primary survey, the annual number of patients seeking medical care, that were treated with shunt operation, and distribution of the age and gender of the patients were estimated.

In the subsequent secondary survey, the detailed clinical epidemiological features of the registered iNPH patients were investigated.

The content of the secondary survey form was as follows: (1) patient attribution, (2) diagnostic level, (3) estimated onset date and age, (4) development in relatives or persons living with, (5) initial symptom, (6) complications, (7) clinical symptoms (throughout the course), (8) imaging findings (magnetic resonance imaging (MRI) of the head including the Evans index as an index of ventricular enlargement: the ratio of the maximum width of the frontal horns of the lateral ventricles and maximal internal diameter of skull at the same level employed in axial MRI images) [6–8, 21], (9) other test findings, (10) treatment (centering shunt operation: ventriculo-peritoneal shunt (VP shunt), ventriculo-atrial shunt (VA shunt), or lumbo-peritoneal shunt (LP shunt) when passage of cerebrospinal fluid is favorable), and (11) outcome.

Accounting for the selection rate and response rate to the survey, we estimated the total number of patients seeking medical care according to the following formula: the estimated total numbers of patients (=reported number of patients/selection rate response rate) = reported number of patients/ (number of reporting departments/number of total departments). Additionally, the 95% confidence interval (CI) was calculated with an assumption of multinominal hypergeometric distribution [19, 20].

$$\text{The estimated total numbers of patients} = \frac{\text{reported number of patients}}{\text{selection rate} \times \text{response rate}}$$

6.5.2 *Results of the Nationwide Survey*

In the primary survey, 4220 sites were extracted from a total of 14,089 sites (university hospital: 459, regular hospital: 13,582, special stratified hospital: 48), and the epidemiological survey was performed using postal mail. Formal replies were sent from 1804 departments, and the response rate was 42.7%. This rate is not high, but similar to those in other reports [19, 20] securing the minimum level.

In the primary survey, 3079 patients met the diagnostic criteria of iNPH, and 1815 patients were treated with shunt operation. As shown in Table 6.2, the values determined in the primary survey were applied in the formula introduced in Methods. The estimated number of iNPH patients who visited medical institution in 2012 was 12,900 (95% Confidence Interval (CI): 10,000–15,800). Based on this, the crude prevalence based on the population of Japanese in 2012 was estimated to be about 10.2 per 100,000 people. The crude prevalence of iNPH in 70–79-year-old and 80-year-old or older people in 2012 were 51.3/100,000 and 50.7/100,000, respectively.

The number of iNPH patients treated with shunt operation in this survey was 6700 (95% CI: 4800–8600). Not all patients were covered by this survey because it was a nationwide hospital-based study in which patients who did not visit a hospital throughout the year were not included, so that the values were estimates to the last, and the number of patients may be larger. Therefore, although the prevalence was lower than the reported prevalence of other neurodegenerative diseases, such as Parkinson disease (180 in 100,000 people) [22], the survey clarified the presence of a considerable number of patients. The onset age distribution peaked in the 70s in both sexes as shown in Fig. 6.1, showing that iNPH is a geriatric disease frequently noted in the golden aged population in their 70s or older. The second highest incidence was above 30% in 80s, and the incidence was 15% or lower in 60s. Regarding sex difference, no particular difference was noted in the age, clarifying that subjective symptoms of iNPH develop in the mid-70s leading to visiting a medical institution.

Table 6.2 The estimated number of iNHP patients during 2013

	The estimated number of cases that meet the diagnostic criteria of iNPH	The estimated numbers of cases performed shunt operation
Estimated number of patients (95% confidence interval)	12,900(10,000–15,800)	6700(4800–8600)

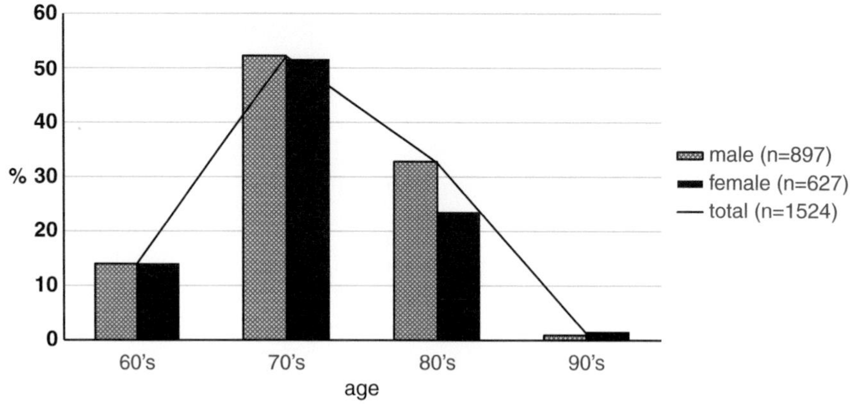

Fig. 6.1 Age distribution of the subjects at the time of diagnosis. The age distribution of registered iNPH patients at the time of definite diagnosis is presented. Analysis is based on the subjects whose age at the time of diagnosis was available. Patients in their 70s accounted for more than 50% of all registrants, being the peak of onset time of this disease. The number of patients in their 80s was the second highest, accounting for more than 30%, and the rate of onset time in 60s was lower than 15%. No characteristic or difference to be mentioned was noted in the age distribution between the sexes

Important findings of the attribution and clinical characteristics concerning classification of diagnostic levels, state of treatment, and shunt operation of the iNPH patients in the secondary survey are summarized in Table 6.3. The replies to the secondary survey of 1524 patients (897 males and 627 females) were valid (Table 6.3). Neurosurgery and neurology departments accounted for 90% of physicians in charge of iNPH treatment, reflecting the disease characteristics of gait disturbance and impaired cognitive function, but a specific number of patients were outpatients of neuropsychiatry and general internal medicine departments because mental symptoms and complaints related to geriatric internal medicine appear as the symptoms progress. Medical cooperation in consideration of comorbidities, accurate diagnostic criteria, and activity enlightening the treatment guidelines may be necessary.

The most frequent diagnostic level was definite iNPH and 799 patients (52.4%) were classified in this level, followed by possible iNPH in 394 (25.8%) and probable iNPH in 267 (17.5%). Since definite iNPH was diagnosed in patients treated with shunt operation for iNPH based on the guidelines, more than half of the patients received active surgical treatment. The remaining half of the patients may have included patients in preparation for surgery or for whom surgical treatment was considered. A prospective survey including education activity, such as how to lead to appropriate selection of shunting, and improvement of treatment skill of attending physicians at outpatient clinics, may be necessary.

The most frequent initial symptom on the first examination was gait disturbance and it was observed in 49.5%, followed by cognitive impairment observed in 15.7%. However, all three features were noted only in 12.1%, clarifying that patients not

Table 6.3 Distribution of clinical background factors

variables	All patients	stratified by gender	
		Male	Female
	$n = 1524$ (100%)	$n = 897$(58.5%)	$n = 627$(40.7%)
	n(%)	n(%)	n(%)
Average age during the prognosis in iNPH			
Age at estimated onset (y.o.)	74.9 ± 7.0 y.o.	74.9 ± 6.7y.o.	74.8 ± 7.5 y.o.
Age at diagnosis (y.o.)	75.5 ± 8.6 y.o.	76.4 ± 6.9 y.o.	76.3 ± 7.3 y.o.
Age of shunt operation (y.o.)	76.4 ± 7.0 y.o.	76.8 ± 8.9 y.o.	76.9 ± 8.0 y.o.
Regular clinical departments in iNPH			
Neurosurgery	1179(77.4%)	685(76.4%)	494(78.8%)
Neurology	262(17.2%)	168(18.7%)	94(15.0%)
Psychology	60(3.9%)	32(3.6%)	28(4.5%)
General medicine	19(1.2%)	10(1.1%)	9(1.4%)
Others	4(0.3%)	2(0.2%)	2(0.3%)
Diagnostic classification			
Possible iNPH	394(25.8%)	223(24.9%)	171(27.3%)
Probable iNPH	267(17.5%)	165(18.4%)	102(16.3%)
Definite iNPH	799(52.4%)	475(53.0%)	324(51.7%)
Unknown	64(4.2%)	34(3.8%)	30(4.8%)
Initial symptoms at 1st visit(multiple answers allowed)			
1. Gait disturbance	755(49.5%)	474(52.8%)[b]	281(44.8%)
2. Cognitive impairment	240(15.7%)	127(14.2%)	113(18.0%)[a]
3. Urinary incontinence	22(1.4%)	9(1.0%)	13(2.1%)
1 + 2 + 3.	185(12.1%)	112(12.5%)	73(11.6%)
Other, unknown	150(9.8%)	84(9.4%)	66(10.5%)
Comorbidity			
Hypertension	609(40.0%)	383(42.7%)[b]	226(36.0%)
Diabetes mellitus	272(17.8%)	185(12.1%)	87(13.9%)[b]
Alzheimer disease	225(14.8%)	129(14.4%)	96(15.3%)
Hyperlipidemia	206(13.5%)	116(12.9%)	89(14.2%)
Lumbar spondylosis	154(10.1%)	85(9.5%)	69(11.0%)
Malignancy	82(5.4%)	54(6.0%)	28(4.0%)
Cervical spondylosis	49(3.2%)	31(3.5%)	18(2.9%)
Shunt treatment			
Shunt operation(+)	1004(65.9%)	594(66.2%)	410(65.4%)
VP shunt (% of operation)	434(43.2%)	248(41.8%)	186(45.4%)
LP shunt (% of operation)	553(55.1%)	334(56.2%)	219(53.4%)
VA shunt (% of operation)	17(1.7%)	12(2.0%)	5(1.2%)
No shunting	464(30.4%)	271(30.2%)	193(30.8%)
Operation unknown, not filled in	56(3.7%)	32(3.6%)	24(3.8%)
Brain MRI evaluation			
MRI finding(+)	1357(89.0%)	801(89.3%)	556(88.7%)

(continued)

Table 6.3 (continued)

variables	All patients	stratified by gender	
		Male	Female
	$n = 1524$ (100%)	$n = 897$(58.5%)	$n = 627$(40.7%)
	n(%)	n(%)	n(%)
Characteristics of MRI findings			
Evans index >0.3	1278(94.2%)	760(94.5%)	518(93.2%)
Periventricular hyperintensity	902(60.5%)	511(63.8%)	391(70.3%)
Chronic ischemic lesion (diameter > 1.5 cm)	142(10.5%)	103(12.9%)[b]	39(7.0%)
MRI not filled-in, unknown	157(11.0%)	96(10.7%)	71(11.3%)
Family history	7(0.5%)	6(0.7%)	1(0.2%)
Father	1	1	0
Mother	0	0	0
Brother	5	4	1
Sister	1	1	0

VP shunt Ventriculo-peritoneal shunt, *LP shunt* Lumbo-peritoneal shunt, *VA shunt* Ventriculo-atrial shunt, *PPV* programmable pressure valves, *DPV* (fixed) differential pressure valve, *y.o.* years old

[a] $p < 0.05$

[b] $p < 0.01$

necessarily complained of subjective symptoms which were easy to be suspected as iNPH. Gait disturbance as an initial symptom was more frequently noted in males than females. In contrast, cognitive impairment was frequently noted in females, showing a significant difference ($p < 0.05$).

Comorbidities in iNPH have recently been attracting interest and considered important to improve morbidity and long-term outcomes of iNPH patients and consider clinical treatment and management [23, 24]. As shown in Table 6.3, the most frequent comorbidity of iNPH was hypertension and it was noted in 40.0%, followed by diabetes in 17.8%, Alzheimer disease in 14.8%, and hyperlipidemia in 13.5%. Orthopedic diseases, lumbar and cervical spondylosis, were noted in 10.1% and 3.2%, respectively, showing the concomitant presence of these diseases in a certain number of patients. The prevalence of hypertension and diabetes were similar to those in the general elderly population, and no specific characteristic was noted in lifestyle-related diseases in iNPH patients. However, high frequencies of hypertension in iNPH patients [25] and complication by secondary diabetes [26] have been reported. Periventricular hyperintensity reflecting cerebral arteriosclerosis and chronic ischemia were observed on MRI of the head in 60.5%. It is possible that lifestyle-related diseases are involved in iNPH as an aggravating or risk factor. The results of time-series surveys are awaited. In addition, many male iNPH patients were hypertensive compared with female patients, whereas many female iNPH patients were diabetic, and a significance difference was noted in both diseases ($p < 0.05$). No particular tendency to be mentioned was noted in the other lifestyle-related diseases including sex difference. It was clarified that management of comorbidities is also important to treat and prevent aggravation of geriatric disease, iNPH.

Dementia and orthopedic diseases known to cause gait disturbance and impairment of cognitive function were also noted in relatively many iNPH patients in this survey, for which discussion on treatment to be selected and how to handle these comorbidities is necessary. For example, an increase in patients with concomitant mild cognitive impairment (MCI) and iNPH is expected, and a prospective follow-up survey may be necessary with regard to the indication of shunt operation for iNPH patients with concomitant MCI. In Japan, focusing on comorbidities of iNPH, especially, Alzheimer disease, a follow-up registration study (SINPHONI-3) on the efficacy of shunt operation for iNPH patients with Alzheimer disease compared with that for patients without Alzheimer disease is being prepared. It is planned to start in 2018 and the results will be paid attention to.

There are three treatment methods: ventriculo-peritoneal shunt (VP shunt), ventriculo-atrial shunt (VA shunt), or lumbo-peritoneal shunt (LP shunt) for cases with favorable passage of cerebrospinal fluid without spinal canal stenosis. As shown in Table 6.3, LP shunt (55.1%) was the first-choice for iNPH patients, and the second was VP shunt, applied in 43.2%. These shunt operations were the current main treatments. Both VP and LP shunts were effective in more than 80%, and the course of patients treated with LP shunt was favorable in more than 90% (data not shown). Previously, V-P shunt operation was the main stream of iNPH treatment, but it has a risk of damaging the brain because a tube is inserted into the brain. This survey clarified that LP shunt has been increasingly applied as the first-choice because the shunt can be placed without puncturing the brain parenchyma in this procedure, being low-invasive. LP shunt may be increasingly selected for elderly iNPH patients in the future. These results may have reflected that consideration of selecting either LP or VP shunt in the same line in consideration of the age, patient's request, and presence or absence of concomitant spinal cord lesions will be generalized [14].

The finding of this survey especially worth mentioning is the presence of familial iNPH at a certain rate, as shown in the lowest row in Table 6.3. It has recently been reported that the clinical symptoms described above overlap, being likely to be promoted and manifested in the early stage [27, 28]. It is possible that iNPH is a multifactorial disease including genes [29]. Genetic epidemiological research by genome-wide association study (GWAS) may be necessary.

6.6 The Meanings Clarified by the Results of Epidemiological Survey: Comparison with Reports on iNPH from Japan and Other Countries

We performed world's first nationwide epidemiologic survey of iNPH and clarified epidemiological information, sex, and clinical characteristics by the classification of diagnostic level of presumed patients. The cause of iNPH is regarded as idiopathic, but it is possible that new background factors will be identified. Comprehensive treatment strategy in consideration of the results of this epidemiological survey is necessary for patients with iNPH characterized by development at an elderly age in 70s or older, and utilization of the results of this survey as basic data for early discovery, treatment, and preventive measures is expected for this intractable disease. Revision of the guidelines for this disease including the survey findings is now underway.

Reports on main epidemiological studies on iNPH from Japan and other countries are listed in Table 6.2, in which the studies are roughly divided into hospital-based and population-based based on the survey method. Although it is natural that the results and data vary depending on the method, target, and year of survey as shown in Table 6.2, reports describing the prevalence and incidence were selected. In Japan, a study on the frequency of iNPH based on several population-based studies has been reported. Hiraoka et al. [30] reported that the prevalence of MRI-supported possible iNPH (suspected iNPH) was 2.9%, Iseki et al. reported 0.4–0.5% [31, 32], Tanaka et al. reported 1.4% [29], and Nakashita et al. reported 2.8% [33], clarifying that iNPH is present at a specific rate, being not rare among geriatric diseases, and the frequency is relatively high. However, the data were collected within a specific region and limited in all these previous reports. Accordingly, the data varies among the reports and the findings do not represent nationwide epidemiological information, such as the number of patients in Japan.

Regarding the annual number of treated patients, the incidence in hospital-based surveys was 1–10/100,000 [9, 34–38], and the prevalence was 10/100,000 [9], whereas in the population-based surveys, the incidence was 120/100,000 [32, 34], showing variation. In the percentage, the prevalence rate was 0.9% in a hospital-based survey [39] and 0.2–2.9% in population-based surveys [29–33, 40], also showing variation.

Variation of the data among countries may have reflected the racial characteristics and medical circumstances in the countries. In addition, various factors are considered, such as variation in the diagnostic criteria and the level of awareness in medical practice. Furthermore, the main body of the population-based surveys was MRI and consultation because it utilized medical check-ups of general residents in the communities, and many cases not examined by cerebrospinal fluid test, tap test, or shunt operation, which are necessary to make a definite diagnosis, may have been included. Thus, the prevalence and morbidity were higher in many population-based than hospital-based studies. It is desirable to utilize the data and values for epidemiological studies on iNPH in each country after fully understanding these conditions.

A retrospective study on iNPH using a health insurance-database has been reported from Germany in 2016 [41], in which the incidence of iNPH was 1.36/100,000/year, being lower than those in the previous hospital-based and population-based studies. Although this was not closely discussed in the report, this may have reflected deviation between the number of actually treated patients and total number of iNPH patients because in diseases for which no internal medical treatment is available and treatment is either surgical shunt operation or course observation with conservative treatment, such as iNPH, patients followed at outpatient clinics or overlooked are present in a certain number. Therefore, although descriptive and analytic epidemiology through a nationwide epidemiological survey is useful, the data should be carefully interpreted because the values may vary among survey reports.

6.7 Characteristics and Points of Attention of Hospital-Based and Population-Based Epidemiological Surveys

Generally, the advantages of the national-level hospital-based epidemiological survey method include the following points: Nationwide tendency can be observed, the findings are not influenced by locality (understanding of disease and distribution of population), a large number of samples can be collected, and consideration of migration and characteristics of the population is not necessary. On the other hand, the points of attention are as follows: The measurement method and treatment standardization may not be completely the same among medical institutions, reducing the accuracy of registered cases, overlapping patients visiting several medical institutions are included, much labor is necessary, and comparison of the morbidity and prevalence with those in other epidemiological surveys should be carefully performed.

Previous surveys performed in many regions were population-based or community-based epidemiological studies, and the characteristic is sampling related to general population defined by the geopolitical boundary. Since the survey is community-based, the survey acceptance rate and follow-up rate increase, facilitating a highly accurate study. The points of attention are as follows: It is necessary to check whether the surveyed population is representative samples, i.e., whether samples are unbiased, in consideration of the characteristics of nationwide population (sociodemographic characteristics, such as the sex, age, and schooling history, health level, and characteristics of community-dwelling elderly), a sufficient number of registrants cannot be collected when the disease is rare, and accurate investigation of new development is difficult when the disease is not rare or acute.

6.8 Conclusion

Through the survey of an intractable disease, iNPH, the importance of descriptive epidemiology and analytic epidemiology of intractable diseases was discussed with regard to the significance, methodology, and points of attention of the nationwide survey that we experienced, with introduction of reports from Japan and other countries. After the guidelines for treatment of iNPH were established, new epidemiological information has been accumulated in Japan. In the present nationwide epidemiologic survey, 13,000 iNPH patients were treated per year in Japan. If iNPH is not overlooked and it is appropriately diagnosed and properly treated with cerebrospinal fluid shunt operation, a long-term treatment effect can be achieved. The clinical characteristics of iNPH, current diagnostic method at medical practice sites, and selection of treatment were clarified, which may facilitate appropriate diagnosis and rapid designing of a treatment strategy. In addition, hypertension, diabetes, Alzheimer disease, and orthopedic diseases were observed as comorbidities of iNPH, and the characteristics due to sex differences were also observed. The data collected by this study are expected to be utilized to elucidate the mechanism related to the fundamental cause and pathology of iNPH as a treatable geriatric disease.

Finally, it should be emphasized that planning of guideline preparation aiming at standardization of diagnosis and treatment of iNPH greatly contributed to promotion of subsequent epidemiological study. For various intractable diseases, not limited to iNPH, data accumulation by country and race is necessary, and returning the descriptive and analytic epidemiological information of these to medical practice sites and patients may be important for the field of clinical epidemiology.

Funding Information The Ministry of Health, Labour and Welfare of Japan (2014-Nanchi-General-052).

References

1. Adams RD, Fisher CM, Hakim S, Ojemann RG, Sweet WH. Symptomatic occult hydrocephalus with "normal" cerebrospinal-fluid pressure. A treatable syndrome. N Engl J Med. 1965;273:117–26. https://doi.org/10.1056/NEJM196507152730301.
2. Hakim S, Adams RD. The special clinical problem of symptomatic hydrocephalus with normal cerebrospinal fluid pressure. Observations on cerebrospinal fluid hydrodynamics. J Neurol Sci. 1965;2:307–27.
3. Collmann H, Sorensen N, Krauss J. Hydrocephalus in craniosynostosis: a review. Childs Nerv Syst. 2005;21:902–12. https://doi.org/10.1007/s00381-004-1116-y.
4. Gallia GL, Rigamonti D, Williams MA. The diagnosis and treatment of idiopathic normal pressure hydrocephalus. Nat Clin Pract Neurol. 2006;2:375–81. https://doi.org/10.1038/ncpneuro0237.
5. Bakker SL, Boon AJ, Wijnhoud AD, Dippel DW, Delwel EJ, Koudstaal PJ. Cerebral hemodynamics before and after shunting in normal pressure hydrocephalus. Acta Neurol Scand. 2002;106:123–7. https://doi.org/10.1034/j.1600-0404.2002.01329.
6. Marmarou A, Black P, Bergsneider M, Klinge P, Relkin N. Guidelines for management of idiopathic normal pressure hydrocephalus: progress to date. Acta Neurochir Suppl. 2005;95:237–40.
7. Mori E, Ishikawa M, Kato T, Kazui H, Miyake H, Miyajima M, Nakajima M, Hashimoto M, Kuriyama N, Tokuda T, Ishii K, Kaijima M, Hirata Y, Saito M, Arai H. Guidelines for management of idiopathic normal pressure hydrocephalus: second edition. Neurol Med Chir (Tokyo). 2012;52:775–809. https://doi.org/10.2176/nmc.52.775.
8. Relkin N, Marmarou A, Klinge P, Bergsneider M, Black PM. Diagnosing idiopathic normal-pressure hydrocephalus. Neurosurgery. 2005;57(3 Suppl):S4–16.
9. Kuriyama N, Miyajima M, Nakajima M, Kurosawa M, Fukushima W, Watanabe Y, Ozaki E, Hirota Y, Tamakoshi A, Mori E, Kato T, Tokuda T, Urae A, Arai H. Nationwide hospital-based

survey of idiopathic normal pressure hydrocephalus in Japan: epidemiological and clinical characteristics. Brain Behav. 2017;7:e00635. https://doi.org/10.1002/brb3.635.
10. Ishikawa M, Hashimoto M, Kuwana N, Mori E, Miyake H, Wachi A, Takeuchi T, Kazui H, Koyama H. Guidelines for management of idiopathic normal pressure hydrocephalus. Neurol Med Chir (Tokyo). 2008;48(Suppl):S1–23. https://doi.org/10.2176/nmc.48.S1.
11. Marmarou A, Young HF, Aygok GA, Sawauchi S, Tsuji O, Yamamoto T, Dunbar J. Diagnosis and management of idiopathic normal-pressure hydrocephalus; a prospective study in 151 patients. J Neurosurg. 2005;102:987–97.
12. Woodworth GF, McGirt MJ, Williams MA, Rigamonti D. Cerebrospinal fluid drainage and dynamics in the diagnosis of normal pressure hydrocephalus. Neurosurgery. 2009;64:919–25. https://doi.org/10.1227/01.NEU.0000341902.44760.10.
13. Hashimoto M, Ishikawa M, Mori E, Kuwana N. Diagnosis of idiopathic normal pressure hydrocephalus is supported by MRI-based scheme: a prospective cohort study. Cerebrospinal Fluid Res. 2010;7:18. https://doi.org/10.1186/1743-8454-7-18.
14. Kazui H, Miyajima M, Mori E, Ishikawa M. Lumboperitoneal shunt surgery for idiopathic normal pressure hydrocephalus (SINPHONI-2): an open-label randomised trial. Lancet Neurol. 2015;14:585–94. https://doi.org/10.1016/S1474-4422(15)00046-0.
15. Johanson C, McMillan P, Tavares R, Spangenberger A, Duncan J, Silverberg G, et al. Homeostatic capabilities of the choroid plexus epithelium in Alzheimer's disease. Cerebrospinal Fluid Res. 2004;3:1. https://doi.org/10.1186/1743-8454-1-3.
16. Klinge P, Hellstrom P, Tans J, Wikkelso C. One-year outcome in the European multicentre study on iNPH. Acta Neurol Scand. 2012;126:145–53. https://doi.org/10.1111/j.1600-0404.2012.01676.x.
17. Klinge PM. Idiopathic normal pressure hydrocephalus--neurosurgical management of dementia! Med Health R I. 2012;95:86–7.
18. Kito Y, Kazui H, Kubo Y, Yoshida T, Takaya M, Wada T, Nomura K, Hashimoto M, Ohkawa S, Miyake H, Ishikawa M, Takeda M. Neuropsychiatric symptoms in patients with idiopathic normal pressure hydrocephalus. Behav Neurol. 2009;21:165–74. https://doi.org/10.3233/BEN-2009-0233.
19. Fukushima W, Fujioka M, Kubo T, Tamakoshi A, Nagai M, Hirota Y. Nationwide epidemiologic survey of idiopathic osteonecrosis of the femoral head. Clin Orthop Relat Res. 2010;468:2715–24. https://doi.org/10.1007/s11999-010-1292-x.
20. Nakamura Y, Matsumoto T, Tamakoshi A, Kawamura T, Seino Y, Kasuga M, Yanagawa H, Ohno Y. Prevalence of idiopathic hypoparathyroidism and pseudohypoparathyroidism in Japan. J Epidemiol. 2000;10:29–33. https://doi.org/10.2188/jea.10.29.
21. Sasaki M, Honda S, Yuasa T, Iwamura A, Shibata E, Ohba H. Narrow CSF space at high convexity and high midline areas in idiopathic normal pressure hydrocephalus detected by axial and coronal MRI. Neuroradiology. 2008;50:117–22. https://doi.org/10.1007/s00234-007-0318-x.
22. Yamawaki M, Kusumi M, Kowa H, Nakashima K. Changes in prevalence and incidence of Parkinson's disease in Japan during a quarter of a century. Neuroepidemiology. 2009;32:263–9. https://doi.org/10.1159/000201565.
23. Andren K, Wikkelso C, Tisell M, Hellstrom P. Natural course of idiopathic normal pressure hydrocephalus. J Neurol Neurosurg Psychiatry. 2014;85:806–10. https://doi.org/10.1136/jnnp-2013-306117.
24. Malm J, Graff-Radford NR, Ishikawa M, Kristensen B, Leinonen V, Mori E, Owler BK, Tullberg M, Williams MA, Relkin NR. Influence of comorbidities in idiopathic normal pressure hydrocephalus - research and clinical care. A report of the ISHCSF task force on comorbidities in INPH. Fluids Barriers CNS. 2013;10:22. https://doi.org/10.1186/2045-8118-10-22.
25. Krauss JK, Regel JP, Vach W, Droste DW, Borremans JJ, Mergner T. Vascular risk factors and arteriosclerotic disease in idiopathic normal-pressure hydrocephalus of the elderly. Stroke. 1996;27:24–9. https://doi.org/10.1161/01.STR.27.1.24.
26. Jacobs L. Diabetes mellitus in normal pressure hydrocephalus. J Neurol Neurosurg Psychiatry. 1977;40:331–5. https://doi.org/10.1136/jnnp.40.4.331.

27. McGirr A, Cusimano MD. Familial aggregation of idiopathic normal pressure hydrocephalus: novel familial case and a family study of the NPH triad in an iNPH patient cohort. J Neurol Sci. 2012;321:82–8. https://doi.org/10.1016/j.jns.2012.07.062.
28. Takahashi Y, Kawanami T, Nagasawa H, Iseki C, Hanyu H, Kato T. Familial normal pressure hydrocephalus (NPH) with an autosomal-dominant inheritance: a novel subgroup of NPH. J Neurol Sci. 2011;308:149–51. https://doi.org/10.1016/j.jns.2011.06.018.
29. Tanaka N, Yamaguchi S, Ishikawa H, Ishii H, Meguro K. Prevalence of possible idiopathic normal-pressure hydrocephalus in Japan: the Osaki-Tajiri project. Neuroepidemiology. 2009;32:171–5. https://doi.org/10.1159/000186501.
30. Hiraoka K, Meguro K, Mori E. Prevalence of idiopathic normal-pressure hydrocephalus in the elderly population of a Japanese rural community. Neurol Med Chir. 2008;48:197–9. https://doi.org/10.1186/1743-8454-7-18.
31. Iseki C, Kawanami T, Nagasawa H, Wada M, Koyama S, Kikuchi K, Arawaka S, Kurita K, Daimon M, Mori E, Kato T. Asymptomatic ventriculomegaly with features of idiopathic normal pressure hydrocephalus on MRI (AVIM) in the elderly: a prospective study in a Japanese population. J Neurol Sci. 2009;277:54–7. https://doi.org/10.1016/j.jns.2008.10.004.
32. Iseki C, Takahashi Y, Wada M, Kawanami T, Adachi M, Kato T. Incidence of idiopathic normal pressure hydrocephalus (iNPH): a 10-year follow-up study of a rural community in Japan. J Neurol Sci. 2014;339:108–12. https://doi.org/10.1016/j.jns.2014.01.033.
33. Nakashita S, Wada-Isoe K, Uemura Y, Tanaka K, Yamamoto M, Yamawaki M, Nakashima K. Clinical assessment and prevalence of parkinsonism in Japanese elderly people. Acta Neurol Scand. 2016;133:373–9. https://doi.org/10.1111/ane.12472.
34. Brean A, Eide PK. Prevalence of probable idiopathic normal pressure hydrocephalus in a Norwegian population. Acta Neurol Scand. 2008;118:48–53. https://doi.org/10.1111/j.1600-0404.2007.00982.x.
35. Klassen BT, Ahlskog JE. Normal pressure hydrocephalus: how often does the diagnosis hold water? Neurology. 2011;77:1119–25. https://doi.org/10.1212/WNL.0b013e31822f02f5.
36. Tisell M, Höglund M, Wikkelsø C. National and regional incidence of surgery for adult hydrocephalus in Sweden. Acta Neurol Scand. 2005;112:72–5. https://doi.org/10.1111/j.1600-0404.2005.00451.x.
37. Vanneste J, Augustijn P, Dirven C, Tan WF, Goedhart ZD. Shunting normal-pressure hydrocephalus: do the benefits outweigh the risks? A multicenter study and literature review. Neurology. 1992;42:54–9.
38. Brean A, Fredø HL, Sollid S, Müller T, Sundstrøm T, Eide PK. Five-year incidence of surgery for idiopathic normal pressure hydrocephalus in Norway. Acta Neurol Scand. 2009;120:314–6. https://doi.org/10.1111/j.1600-0404.2009.01250.
39. Muangpaisan W, Petcharat C, Srinonprasert V. Prevalence of potentially reversible conditions in dementia and mild cognitive impairment in a geriatric clinic. Geriatr Gerontol Int. 2012;12:59–64. https://doi.org/10.1111/j.1447-0594.2011.00728.x.
40. Jaraj D, Rabiei K, Marlow T, Jensen C, Skoog I, Wikkelso C. Prevalence of idiopathic normal-pressure hydrocephalus. Neurology. 2014;82:1449–54. https://doi.org/10.1212/WNL.0000000000000342.
41. Lemcke J, Stengel D, Stockhammer F, Guthoff C, Rohde V, Meier U. Nationwide incidence of normal pressure hydrocephalus (NPH) assessed by insurance claim data in Germany. Open Neurol J. 2016;10:15–24. https://doi.org/10.2174/1874205X01610010015.

Chapter 7
Case-Control Study of Idiopathic Pulmonary Fibrosis in Japan

Yoshihiro Miyake

Abstract With regard to risk factors for idiopathic pulmonary fibrosis (IPF), the results from a case-control study of a Japanese population were shown. Included in the study were 104 patients of IPF, aged 40 years or over, who had been diagnosed within the previous 2 years, in accordance with the most recent criteria. Control subjects, aged 40 years or over, consisted of 56 hospitalized patients diagnosed as having acute bacterial pneumonia and four outpatients with the common cold. Exposure to metal dust was related to an approximately tenfold increased risk of IPF. A significant increased risk of IPF was observed for smokers with 20.0–39.9 pack-years. Intake levels of saturated fatty acids and meat were independently related to an increased risk of IPF. Consumption of fruit in the second and third quartiles was associated with a statistically significant reduced risk of IPF. Having a child with a history of allergic rhinitis was significantly related to an increased risk of IPF. Epidemiological investigations regarding gene–environment interaction affecting the risk of IPF are required.

Keywords Case-control study · Japan · Idiopathic pulmonary fibrosis · Risk factor

7.1 Introduction

Idiopathic pulmonary fibrosis (IPF) is characterized by progressive scarring of the lung parenchyma, which leads to dyspnea and declining pulmonary function and eventually to respiratory failure. The median survival after diagnosis of IPF is 3–5 years [1]. The heterogeneity in radiological and histopathological appearances, rate of progression, and treatment response observed in individuals with IPF suggests that fibrosis arises as a consequence of multiple co-activated pathogenic

Y. Miyake
Department of Epidemiology and Preventive Medicine, Ehime University Graduate School of Medicine, Ehime, Japan
e-mail: miyake.yoshihiro.ls@ehime-u.ac.jp

M. Washio, G. Kobashi (eds.), *Epidemiological Studies of Specified Rare and Intractable Disease*, Current Topics in Environmental Health and Preventive Medicine, https://doi.org/10.1007/978-981-13-1096-6_7

pathways, all of which are influenced by complex interactions between endogenous and environmental factors [2]. Smoking has long been described as a prevalent risk factor for the development of IPF [2]. Some other environmental and occupational exposures, including wood, mineral, and metal dusts, agriculture, and livestock, have also been associated with IPF [2].

In this chapter, using data from the Japan Idiopathic Pulmonary Fibrosis Study, the results from a case-control study of a Japanese population were shown [3–6].

7.2 A Case-Control Study in Japan

7.2.1 Study Population

Eligible cases aged 40 years or over who were within 2 years of having been diagnosed with IPF were identified among 21 collaborating hospitals and their 29 affiliated hospitals during the period from 1 June to 30 November 2001. The diagnosis of IPF by the collaborating respiratory disease specialists was based on clinical history, clinical examination, and high-resolution computerized tomography (HRCT) of the chest. Results of video-assisted thoracoscopic lung biopsy transbronchial lung biopsy and/or bronchoalveolar lavage, corresponding to the international consensus statement on IPF of the American Thoracic Society and the European Respiratory Society [7], were also used when available, either alone or in combination, to assist diagnosis. All cases had basal fine crackles through auscultation and predominantly peripheral, subpleural, bibasal fine reticular shadows and/or honeycombing, occasionally with traction bronchiectasis and bronchiolectasis on HRCT. There was no evidence of either coexisting collagen-vascular disease or history of known occupational exposure to agents that might produce a clinical picture similar to that of IPF in any of the cases. The physicians in charge asked eligible patients to participate in this study, and 104 patients were cooperative in answering the questionnaires while three patients refused. Control subjects, aged 40 years or over and without prior respiratory diseases, were prospectively selected from individuals who received treatment at the respiratory ward of the 21 collaborating hospitals and their 29 affiliated hospitals during the same time period as the cases. Potential control subjects consisted of 56 hospitalized patients diagnosed as having acute bacterial pneumonia and four outpatients with common colds. Only one eligible control subject who was asked to take part in this study by a physician refused to answer the questionnaire.

Controls were not, individually or in larger groups, matched to cases. Few patients with acute infectious or common diseases receive treatment at a specialized medical institution. Of the 21 collaborating hospitals, 14 were university hospitals with doctors who exclusively treated patients with serious illnesses. Thus, 95 of the 104 cases were recruited from the 21 collaborating hospitals and 34 of the 60 controls were selected from 29 hospitals that were affiliated to the collaborating hospitals. Hypertension, hyperlipidemia, coronary heart disease, diabetes mellitus, tuberculosis, asthma, atopic dermatitis, and allergic rhinitis (including cedar pollinosis) were defined as present when subjects had been under drug treatment, or, in the case of diabetes mellitus, if they were receiving dietary therapy. Hepatitis C virus was considered present if the subject had been diagnosed by a physician as having hepatitis C virus or being its carrier. A child's history of asthma, atopic dermatitis, and allergic rhinitis (including cedar pollinosis) was considered to be confirmed if one or more children of the study subject had been treated for these conditions with medications at some time since birth. Occupational exposure was defined as present if the subject had been exposed to any of eight specific occupational agents (metal, wood, asbestos, coal, stone and sand, solvents, pesticide, or chalk) ten or more hours per week for more than 1 year. All study subjects gave their fully informed consent in writing.

The study subjects were originally restricted to males, but included in the analysis were 10 female cases and five female controls whose treatment was provided at six of the collaborating hospitals and one affiliated hospital.

7.2.2 Measurement

A set of two self-administered questionnaires was handed to cases and controls by physicians. The subjects filled out the questionnaires and mailed them to the data management center. A telephone interview was conducted by a trained research technician to complete missing or illogical data. One of the self-administered questionnaires elicited information on age, sex, type of job held for the longest period of time, exposure to 13 specific occupational agents, smoking habits, molds in the house, indoor domestic pets, and residential municipality. Employment data focused on type of job held for the longest period of time during the subject's work life and years of exposure were requested regarding the job and occupational agents, respectively. Occupational agents were defined as present if the subject reported >10 h of exposure per week. Neither the questionnaire nor a telephone interview requested a full occupational history or gave any information to help responders recall possible exposures to occupational agents that they may otherwise have overlooked in relation to their particular occupation.

The other self-administered questionnaire was a validated self-administered dietary history questionnaire that was used to assess dietary habits over a period of 1 month [8, 9]. The structure and validity of the questionnaire are described in detail elsewhere [8, 9]. Energy-adjusted intake by the residual method was used for the analyses [10].

7.2.3 Statistical Analysis

Jobs held for the longest period of time were coded using the Japanese Standard Occupational Classification and stratified into 11 major groups (professional and technical; managers and officials; clerical and related fields; sales; service; protective service; farming, fishing and forestry; transport and communication; production;

materials handling; and construction and extraction). Included in this analysis were eight specific occupational agents to which three or more subjects had been exposed for more than a year. Intake of foods and nutrients under study was categorized at quartile points. Age was classified into four categories (<50, 50–59, 60–69, and 70+ years); region into five (Kanto-Koshinetsu, Tokai, Kinki, Chugoku-Shikoku, and Kyushu); cigarette smoking into three (never smoked, former smoker, and current smoker); pack-years of smoking into five (none, 0–19.9, 20.0–39.9, 40.0–59.9, and 60.0+); and residential municipality into two (city and town or village). Multiple logistic regression analysis was used to estimate the adjusted ORs and 95% confidence intervals (CIs) of IPF for single factors with adjustment for age, sex, and region. The reference category for all occupational factors, molds in the house, and indoor domestic pets was based on the comparison of those exposed to a single agent with all those unexposed, including potential subjects who were exposed to other etiologic factors. All computations were performed using version 8.2 of the SAS software package (SAS Institute, Inc., Cary, NC, USA).

7.3 Results

Dyspnea on exertion was present at enrollment in 84 of the 104 cases (80.8%). The median (90% central range) of arterial O_2 pressure was 80.2 mmHg (57.2–98.0) and of vital capacity expressed as percent predicted values was 78.0% (42.1–113.5) in cases (Table 7.1).

About 90% of both cases and controls were male (Table 7.2). In comparison with controls, cases were older and had a lower prevalence of residence in Chugoku-Shikoku and never smoking and a higher prevalence of high employment status, occupational exposure, and being overweight.

Table 7.3 presents adjusted ORs and 95% CIs for IPF in relation to occupational factors after controlling for age, sex, and region. None of the occupational groups was related to the risk of IPF with statistical significance, although at least a twofold increase in OR was observed among managers and officials and production workers while there was a less than 0.5-fold decrease in OR among those in clerical and related fields, protective service, and materials handling. Further adjustment for pack-years of smoking slightly strengthened associations with the following two major occupational groups: managers and officials and clerical and related occupations (adjusted ORs were 6.06, 95% CI: 0.97 to 118.6 and 0.42, 95% CI: 0.18 to

Table 7.1 Clinical features of idiopathic pulmonary fibrosis cases

Lung function	Mean	SD	Minimum	Median	Maximum
Arterial O_2 pressure (mmHg)	79.6	11.4	50.0	80.6	102.0
Vital capacity (%, predicted)	77.4	22.0	19.8	77.6	128.0

Arterial O_2 pressure: missing = 8
Vital capacity: missing = 5

Table 7.2 Characteristics of study population

	n (%) or mean (SD)		
Variable	Cases (*n* = 104)	Controls (*n* = 60)	*p* value
Sex (% male)	94 (90.4)	55 (91.7)	0.78
Age (% years)			0.10
<50	3 (2.9)	2 (3.3)	
50–59	16 (15.4)	19 (31.7)	
60–69	56 (53.9)	25 (41.7)	
70+	29 (27.9)	14 (23.3)	
Region (%)			0.21
Kanto-Koshinetsu	57 (54.8)	27 (45.0)	
Tokai	12 (11.5)	10 (16.7)	
Kinki	14 (13.5)	5 (8.3)	
Chugoku-shikoku	4 (3.9)	7 (11.7)	
Kyushu	17 (16.4)	11 (18.3)	
Pack-years of smoking (%)			0.26
Never	20 (19.2)	15 (25.0)	
0 < −19.9	10 (9.6)	11 (18.3)	
20.0–39.9	30 (28.9)	10 (16.7)	
40.0–59.9	29 (27.9)	15 (25.0)	
60.0+	15 (14.4)	9 (15.0)	
High employment status (%)[a]	18 (17.3)	8 (13.3)	0.50
Occupational exposure (%)[b]	33 (31.7)	5 (8.3)	0.0006
Body mass index (kg/m^2)	23.3 (3.1)	21.9 (3.0)	0.005

[a]Subjects considered to have a high employment status were those who were professionals, technical workers, managers or officials for the longest period within their working years
[b]Exposure to metal, wood, asbestos, coal, stone and sand, solvents, pesticide, or chalk 10 or more hours per week for more than 1 year

0.95, respectively). Exposure to any of the eight kinds of dust under study was significantly associated with an increased risk of IPF. In particular, exposure to metal dust was related to an approximately tenfold increased risk of IPF.

Results for environmental factors are shown in Table 7.4. More cases than control subjects were former smokers while current smoking was more prevalent in controls than in cases although differences between groups were not statistically significant. Adjusted OR for comparison of having smoked with never having smoked was 1.91 (95% CI: 0.71 to 5.15). A significant increased risk of IPF was observed for smokers with 20.0–39.9 pack-years, but there was no dose-response association with cumulative consumption of cigarettes. Although not statistically significant, molds in the living room and the presence of indoor hamsters were associated with more than a 50% decreased risk of IPF.

In Table 7.5, adjusted ORs for associations between specific types of dietary fat and IPF are presented. Intake of saturated fatty acids was independently related to an increased risk of IPF after multivariate adjustment: the OR for comparison of the highest with the lowest quartile was 6.26 (95% CI: 1.79 to 24.96; *p* for trend = 0.01).

Table 7.3 Adjusted odds ratios for idiopathic pulmonary fibrosis in relation to occupational factors

Factor	*n* (%)		Adjusted odds ratio[a]	95% confidence interval
	Cases ($n = 102$)	Controls ($n = 59$)		
Job held for the longest period of time				
Professional or technical	9 (8.8)	7 (11.9)	0.71	0.23 to 2.25
Manager or official	9 (8.8)	1 (1.7)	4.26	0.74 to 80.88
Clerical or related occupation	18 (17.7)	18 (30.5)	0.49	0.22 to 1.08
Sales	11 (10.8)	6 (10.2)	1.29	0.44 to 4.18
Service	6 (5.9)	3 (5.1)	1.02	0.23 to 5.46
Protective service	2 (2.0)	3 (5.1)	0.33	0.04 to 2.19
Farming, fishing, or forestry	7 (6.9)	7 (11.9)	0.55	0.16 to 1.89
Transport or communication	4 (3.9)	2 (3.4)	1.10	0.19 to 8.73
Production	18 (17.7)	5 (8.5)	2.56	0.91 to 8.54
Materials handling	2 (2.0)	2 (3.4)	0.46	0.05 to 4.34
Construction or extraction	11 (10.8)	5 (8.5)	1.37	0.42 to 4.44
Occupational agents				
Any dust[b]	33 (32.4)	5 (8.5)	5.61	2.12 to 17.89
Metal	12 (11.8)	1 (1.7)	9.55	1.68 to 181.12
Wood	5 (4.9)	0 (0.0)		
Asbestos	3 (2.9)	0 (0.0)		
Coal	3 (2.9)	0 (0.0)		
Stone or sand	11 (10.8)	4 (6.8)	1.75	0.52 to 7.01
Solvents	4 (3.9)	0 (0.0)		
Pesticides	6 (5.9)	2 (3.4)	1.46	0.30 to 10.61
Chalk	4 (3.9)	0 (0.0)		

[a]Adjusted for age (<50, 50–59, 60–69, or 70+), sex, and region (Kanto-Koshinetsu, Tokai, Kinki, Chugoku-Shikoku, and Kyushu)

[b]Eight cases and 2 controls were exposed to two or more occupational agents

We observed a clear positive association for monounsaturated fatty acids (multivariate OR for comparison of the highest with the lowest quartile = 3.19, 95% CI: 1.06 to 10.14; p for trend = 0.02). For n-6 polyunsaturated fatty acids, a significant positive association was found when comparing the third with the first quartile, but the OR for comparison of the highest with the lowest quartile was slightly above unity (p for trend = 0.20). Intake of n-3 polyunsaturated fatty acids and cholesterol was not statistically significantly associated with the risk of IPF.

We then evaluated the risk of IPF based on intake of high-fat foods (Table 7.6). After adjustment for sex, age, region, pack-years of smoking, employment status, occupational exposure, fruit intake, and body mass index, compared with meat intake in the first quartile, consumption of meat in the second and fourth quartiles

Table 7.4 Adjusted odds ratios for idiopathic pulmonary fibrosis in relation to environmental factors

Factor	*n* (%)		Adjusted odds ratio[a]	95% confidence interval
	Cases (*n* = 102)	Controls (*n* = 59)		
Smoking status				
Never smoked	18 (17.6)	14 (23.7)	1.00	
Former smoker	80 (78.4)	34 (57.6)	2.21	0.82 to 6.04
Current smoker	4 (3.9)	11 (18.6)	0.50	0.10 to 2.24
Pack-years of smoking				
None	18 (17.7)	14 (23.7)	1.00	
0.6–19.9	10 (9.8)	11 (18.6)	0.87	0.25 to 3.10
20.0–39.9	30 (29.4)	10 (17.0)	3.23	1.01 to 10.84
40.0–59.9	29 (28.4)	15 (25.4)	2.22	0.70 to 7.23
60.0+	15 (14.7)	9 (15.3)	1.59	0.46 to 5.64
Molds				
Any place[b]	56 (54.9)	36 (61.0)	0.98	0.48 to 2.01
Living room	5 (4.9)	8 (13.6)	0.36	0.10 to 1.20
Bathroom	51 (50.0)	28 (47.5)	1.38	0.69 to 2.82
Kitchen	12 (11.8)	11 (18.6)	0.61	0.24 to 1.57
Closets	17 (16.7)	9 (15.3)	1.25	0.50 to 3.30
Indoor domestic pets				
Any pets[c]	40 (39.2)	25 (42.4)	0.94	0.47 to 1.86
Birds	17 (16.7)	9 (15.3)	1.16	0.47 to 3.03
Cats	14 (13.7)	8 (13.6)	1.24	0.45 to 3.58
Dogs	15 (14.7)	10 (17.0)	0.85	0.33 to 2.26
Hamsters	2 (2.0)	3 (5.1)	0.27	0.03 to 1.80
Residential municipality				
Village or town	15 (14.7)	12 (20.3)	1.00	
City	87 (85.3)	47 (79.7)	1.35	0.56 to 3.28

[a]Adjusted for age (<50, 50–59, 60–69, or 70+), sex, and region (Kanto-Koshinetsu, Tokai, Kinki, Chugoku-Shikoku, and Kyushu)
[b]Twenty-two cases and 13 controls were exposed to molds in two or more places
[c]Eight cases and 3 controls had two or more types of indoor domestic pets

was associated with a 5.9- and 7.2-fold increased risk of IPF, respectively, while meat consumption in the third quartile had no such statistically significant relationship.

Table 7.7 shows the relation between vegetable, fruit, and cereal consumption and IPF risk. Consumption of fruit in the second and third quartiles was associated with a statistically significant reduced risk of IPF. Although not statistically significant, a beneficial association between soluble fiber intake and IPF was found (Table 7.8).

In Table 7.9, adjusted ORs for associations between selected medical histories and IPF are presented. There was a tendency for an inverse association between

Table 7.5 Odds ratios for idiopathic pulmonary fibrosis by quartiles of specific types of dietary fat

	n (%)		Sex and age adjusted		Multivariate[a]	
Variables[b]	Cases	Controls	Odds ratio	95% CI	Odds ratio	95% CI
Total fat						
Q1 (31.7)	22 (21.2)	19 (31.7)	1.00		1.00	
Q2 (44.8)	23 (22.1)	18 (30.0)	0.96	0.38 to 2.39	1.00	0.32 to 3.11
Q3 (52.3)	31 (29.8)	10 (16.7)	2.33	0.89 to 6.35	2.59	0.79 to 8.85
Q4 (65.5)	28 (26.9)	13 (21.7)	2.02	0.79 to 5.34	2.79	0.93 to 8.69
p for trend			0.05		0.02	
Saturated fatty acids						
Q1 (8.5)	23 (22.1)	18 (30.0)	1.00		1.00	
Q2 (12.4)	22 (21.2)	19 (31.7)	0.79	0.32 to 1.96	0.64	0.20 to 2.03
Q3 (15.3)	24 (23.1)	17 (28.3)	0.92	0.36 to 2.32	0.66	0.22 to 1.93
Q4 (18.9)	35 (33.7)	6 (10.0)	5.50	1.84 to 18.64	6.26	1.79 to 24.96
p for trend			0.007		0.01	
Monounsaturated fatty acids						
Q1 (9.7)	21 (20.2)	20 (33.3)	1.00		1.00	
Q2 (14.8)	25 (24.0)	16 (26.7)	1.37	0.55 to 3.43	1.52	0.50 to 4.71
Q3 (17.5)	30 (28.9)	11 (18.3)	2.49	0.97 to 6.62	4.29	1.30 to 15.20
Q4 (22.9)	28 (26.9)	13 (21.7)	2.38	0.92 to 6.34	3.19	1.06 to 10.14
p for trend			0.04		0.02	
n-3 polyunsaturated fatty acids						
Q1 (1.5)	24 (23.1)	17 (28.3)	1.00		1.00	
Q2 (2.4)	29 (27.9)	12 (20.0)	1.49	0.57 to 3.92	2.14	0.67 to 7.12
Q3 (2.9)	25 (24.0)	16 (26.7)	1.08	0.43 to 2.68	1.74	0.59 to 5.23
Q4 (4.0)	26 (25.0)	15 (25.0)	1.17	0.47 to 2.97	1.72	0.60 to 5.09
p for trend			0.92		0.41	
n-6 polyunsaturated fatty acids						
Q1 (6.1)	25 (24.0)	16 (26.7)	1.00		1.00	
Q2 (9.0)	21 (20.2)	20 (33.3)	0.72	0.29 to 1.79	1.10	0.34 to 3.58
Q3 (10.9)	33 (31.7)	8 (13.3)	2.59	0.96 to 7.44	5.15	1.42 to 20.46
Q4 (14.1)	25 (24.0)	16 (26.7)	1.06	0.42 to 2.72	1.39	0.44 to 4.47
p for trend			0.35		0.20	
Cholesterol						
Q1 (139.2)	24 (23.1)	17 (28.3)	1.00		1.00	
Q2 (220.0)	26 (25.0)	15 (25.0)	1.06	0.41 to 2.72	1.46	0.48 to 4.51
Q3 (290.3)	25 (24.0)	16 (26.7)	0.89	0.35 to 2.29	1.11	0.38 to 3.28
Q4 (418.1)	29 (27.9)	12 (20.0)	1.52	0.59 to 4.01	2.58	0.86 to 8.07
p for trend			0.48		0.15	

CI confidence interval

[a]Adjusted for age, sex, region, pack-years of smoking, employment status, occupational exposure, soluble fiber intake, and body mass index

[b]Quartile medians in grams (except for cholesterol; milligrams) per day adjusted for energy intake using residual methods are given in parentheses

Table 7.6 Odds ratios for idiopathic pulmonary fibrosis by quartiles of intake of selected foods high in fat

	n (%)		Sex and age adjusted		Multivariate[a]	
Variables[b]	Cases	Controls	Odds ratio	95% CI	Odds ratio	95% CI
Meat						
Q1 (15.4)	21 (20.2)	20 (33.3)	1.00		1.00	
Q2 (32.7)	31 (29.8)	10 (16.7)	2.98	1.16 to 8.06	5.90	1.76 to 21.70
Q3 (44.7)	22 (21.2)	19 (31.7)	1.25	0.51 to 3.08	2.11	0.71 to 6.56
Q4 (79.9)	30 (28.9)	11 (18.3)	3.65	1.38 to 10.35	7.19	2.15 to 27.07
p for trend			0.06		0.02	
Eggs						
Q1 (5.4)	24 (23.1)	17 (28.3)	1.00		1.00	
Q2 (14.8)	24 (23.1)	17 (28.3)	0.84	0.32 to 2.15	1.11	0.36 to 3.42
Q3 (25.5)	26 (25.0)	15 (25.0)	1.03	0.40 to 2.65	1.08	0.37 to 3.15
Q4 (47.9)	30 (28.9)	11 (18.3)	1.55	0.58 to 4.22	2.38	0.74 to 8.10
p for trend			0.32		0.19	
Dairy products						
Q1 (14.7)	24 (23.1)	17 (28.3)	1.00		1.00	
Q2 (74.1)	25 (24.0)	16 (26.7)	1.09	0.43 to 2.74	0.83	0.27 to 2.55
Q3 (161.7)	27 (26.0)	14 (23.3)	1.27	0.51 to 3.22	0.80	0.26 to 2.48
Q4 (237.2)	28 (26.9)	13 (21.7)	1.33	0.52 to 3.46	1.32	0.43 to 4.11
p for trend			0.51		0.62	
Fish						
Q1 (34.7)	24 (23.1)	17 (28.3)	1.00		1.00	
Q2 (64.1)	27 (26.0)	14 (23.3)	1.41	0.56 to 3.63	2.38	0.76 to 7.74
Q3 (85.6)	26 (25.0)	15 (25.0)	1.30	0.51 to 3.32	1.62	0.54 to 4.93
Q4 (123.5)	27 (26.0)	14 (23.3)	1.29	0.51 to 3.33	2.12	0.71 to 6.56
p for trend			0.64		0.32	

CI confidence interval

[a]Adjusted for age, sex, region, pack-years of smoking, employment status, occupational exposure, fruit intake, and body mass index

[b]Quartile medians in grams per day adjusted for energy intake using residual methods are given in parentheses

asthma and the risk of IPF: the multivariate OR was 0.22 (95% CI: 0.04 to 1.09). The multivariate OR for a child's history of asthma was 1.82 (95% CI: 0.54 to 7.04), of atopic dermatitis was 0.91 (95% CI: 0.30 to 2.77), and of allergic rhinitis was 2.49 (95% CI: 1.01 to 6.54).

Table 7.7 Odds ratios for idiopathic pulmonary fibrosis by quartiles of vegetable, fruit, and cereal intake

	n (%)		Sex and age adjusted		Multivariate adjusted[a]	
Variables[b]	Cases	Controls	Odds ratio	95% confidence interval	Odds ratio	95% confidence interval
Green and yellow vegetables						
Q1 (32.6)	22 (21.2)	19 (31.7)	1.00		1.00	
Q2 (63.3)	33 (31.7)	8 (13.3)	3.56	1.32 to 10.33	7.06	2.00 to 27.91
Q3 (95.3)	22 (21.2)	19 (31.7)	0.87	0.35 to 2.14	1.02	0.34 to 3.09
Q4 (162.8)	27 (26.0)	14 (23.3)	1.35	0.53 to 3.52	1.62	0.48 to 5.59
p for trend			0.82		0.68	
Other vegetables						
Q1 (81.9)	28 (26.9)	13 (21.7)	1.00		1.00	
Q2 (134.9)	25 (24.0)	16 (26.7)	0.65	0.25 to 1.67	0.61	0.20 to 1.78
Q3 (175.4)	26 (25.0)	15 (25.0)	0.65	0.25 to 1.69	0.59	0.18 to 1.91
Q4 (256.8)	25 (24.0)	16 (26.7)	0.62	0.24 to 1.60	0.77	0.25 to 2.35
p for trend			0.36		0.72	
Fruit						
Q1 (37.9)	33 (31.7)	8 (13.3)	1.00		1.00	
Q2 (108.5)	23 (22.1)	18 (30.0)	0.29	0.10 to 0.80	0.17	0.05 to 0.56
Q3 (181.5)	23 (22.1)	18 (30.0)	0.24	0.08 to 0.66	0.13	0.03 to 0.44
Q4 (312.5)	25 (24.0)	16 (26.7)	0.26	0.08 to 0.75	0.28	0.07 to 1.01
p for trend			0.02		0.06	
Cereals						
Q1 (361.3)	28 (26.9)	13 (21.7)	1.00		1.00	
Q2 (470.5)	29 (27.9)	12 (20.0)	1.00	0.38 to 2.65	0.96	0.30 to 3.02
Q3 (540.7)	27 (26.0)	14 (23.3)	0.75	0.28 to 1.97	0.99	0.31 to 3.12
Q4 (668.5)	20 (19.2)	21 (35.0)	0.42	0.16 to 1.07	0.75	0.21 to 2.64
p for trend			0.06		0.70	

[a]Odds ratios were separately calculated for each dietary variable adjusted for age, sex, region, pack-years of smoking, employment status, occupational exposure, saturated fatty acid intake, and body mass index

[b]Quartile medians in grams per day adjusted for energy intake with the residual methods given in parentheses

Table 7.8 Odds ratios for idiopathic pulmonary fibrosis by quartiles of beta-carotene, vitamins C and E, and fiber intake

	n (%)		Sex and age adjusted		Multivariate adjusted[a]	
Variables[b]	Cases	Controls	Odds ratio	95% confidence interval	Odds ratio	95% confidence interval
Beta-carotene						
Q1 (637.3)	28 (26.9)	13 (21.7)	1.00		1.00	
Q2 (1417.8)	26 (25.0)	15 (25.0)	0.74	0.28 to 1.91	0.93	0.31 to 2.85
Q3 (2258.4)	22 (21.2)	19 (31.7)	0.46	0.17 to 1.16	0.59	0.19 to 1.78
Q4 (3485.8)	28 (26.9)	13 (21.7)	0.81	0.30 to 2.16	1.03	0.32 to 3.32
p for trend			0.46		0.85	
Vitamin C						
Q1 (65.8)	27 (26.0)	14 (23.3)	1.00		1.00	
Q2 (111.6)	28 (26.9)	13 (21.7)	0.77	0.28 to 2.07	1.05	0.32 to 3.38
Q3 (158.7)	25 (24.0)	16 (26.7)	0.54	0.20 to 1.44	0.62	0.19 to 1.97
Q4 (220.9)	24 (23.1)	17 (28.3)	0.49	0.18 to 1.33	0.69	0.20 to 2.40
p for trend			0.13		0.42	
Vitamin E						
Q1 (5.9)	25 (24.0)	16 (26.7)	1.00		1.00	
Q2 (8.0)	28 (26.9)	13 (21.7)	1.28	0.50 to 3.32	1.23	0.38 to 4.04
Q3 (9.3)	26 (25.0)	15 (25.0)	1.05	0.41 to 2.70	0.80	0.23 to 2.70
Q4 (12.0)	25 (24.0)	16 (26.7)	0.93	0.37 to 2.35	0.69	0.21 to 2.19
p for trend			0.78		0.38	
Soluble fiber						
Q1 (1.3)	28 (26.9)	13 (21.7)	1.00		1.00	
Q2 (1.9)	27 (26.0)	14 (23.3)	0.68	0.25 to 1.80	0.54	0.17 to 1.71
Q3 (2.5)	25 (24.0)	16 (26.7)	0.55	0.20 to 1.47	0.56	0.17 to 1.83
Q4 (3.6)	24 (23.1)	17 (28.3)	0.43	0.15 to 1.15	0.36	0.10 to 1.15
p for trend			0.09		0.11	
Insoluble fiber						
Q1 (6.9)	26 (25.0)	15 (25.0)	1.00		1.00	
Q2 (9.4)	28 (26.9)	13 (21.7)	1.16	0.44 to 3.05	0.96	0.31 to 2.90
Q3 (11.4)	25 (24.0)	16 (26.7)	0.68	0.26 to 1.77	0.72	0.22 to 2.24
Q4 (14.5)	25 (24.0)	16 (26.7)	0.61	0.22 to 1.67	0.62	0.18 to 2.05
p for trend			0.22		0.37	

[a]Odds ratios were separately calculated for each dietary variable adjusted for age, sex, region, pack-years of smoking, employment status, occupational exposure, saturated fatty acid intake, and body mass index

[b]Quartile medians in grams (except for beta-carotene and vitamins C and E; milligrams) per day adjusted for energy intake with the residual methods given in parentheses

Table 7.9 Odds ratios for idiopathic pulmonary fibrosis in relation to selected items from personal and child's medical history

	n (%)		Sex and age adjusted		Multivariate adjusted[a]	
Variable	Cases	Controls	Odds ratio	95% confidence interval	Odds ratio	95% confidence interval
Personal history						
Hypertension	28 (26.9)	15 (25.0)	1.00	0.48 to 2.14	0.56	0.23 to 1.35
Hyperlipidemia	10 (9.6)	4 (6.7)	1.63	0.50 to 6.37	1.35	0.34 to 6.39
Coronary disease	10 (9.6)	3 (5.0)	1.58	0.45 to 7.39	1.31	0.32 to 6.76
Diabetes mellitus	13 (12.5)	7 (11.7)	0.95	0.36 to 2.74	1.43	0.46 to 4.76
Hepatitis C virus	7 (6.7)	4 (6.7)	0.85	0.22 to 3.60	0.80	0.15 to 4.27
Tuberculosis	7 (6.7)	9 (15.0)	0.35	0.12 to 1.03	0.58	0.17 to 1.94
Asthma	4 (3.9)	6 (10.0)	0.39	0.09 to 1.48	0.22	0.04 to 1.09
Atopic dermatitis	2 (1.9)	1 (1.7)	1.31	0.12 to 29.99	1.76	0.12 to 46.06
Allergic rhinitis	12 (11.5)	4 (6.7)	1.96	0.62 to 7.58	2.00	0.53 to 9.19
Child's history						
Asthma	12 (11.5)	5 (8.3)	1.56	0.53 to 5.33	1.82	0.54 to 7.04
Atopic dermatitis	9 (8.7)	9 (15.0)	0.56	0.20 to 1.56	0.91	0.30 to 2.77
Allergic rhinitis	30 (28.9)	11 (18.3)	1.94	0.89 to 4.49	2.49	1.01 to 6.54

[a]Adjusted for age, sex, region, pack-years of smoking, employment status, occupational exposure, and body mass index

7.4 Discussion

The present case-control study had methodological advantages. Cases were selected according to the most recent diagnostic criteria and extensive information on potential confounding factors was incorporated. Weaknesses of this study should be borne in mind. Although selection bias in the choice of cases was not likely to have occurred because of the high response rate (only three eligible patients refused), control subjects may not have been representative of the general population from which the cases arose because almost all controls were hospitalized patients with acute bacterial pneumonia. In fact, the prevalence values of hypertension and diabetes mellitus were relatively high in the present study. In a population-based case-control study of acute myocardial infarction in Fukuoka, Japan, the proportions of persons with hypertension and diabetes mellitus, which were considered to be present by the same definition as in this study, were 13% and 10%, respectively, among 260 male controls below 65 years of age, and 21% and 8%, respectively, in 212 male controls aged 65 years or over [11]. The corresponding figures in this study for hypertension and diabetes mellitus were 27% and 10%, respectively, in 30 male controls below 65 years old, and 28% and 16%, respectively, in 25 male controls aged 65 years or over. Our control subjects may have been likely to have had histories of medical conditions such as hypertension and diabetes mellitus. Such a hypothesis would give rise to an underestimation of our results. If acute bacterial pneumonia shared risk factors with IPF, the reported OR would have been underestimated. Eligible control subjects with acute bacterial pneumonia were not likely to arise during the summer months because of seasonal variation in this disease. The ratio of controls to cases was below 1:1 and our investigation did not have a substantial statistical power.

Data on genetic factors were not available in the present case-control study. Common variants (defined as minor allele frequency of >5%) appear to play a role in FIP risk. The most widely replicated risk variant (rs35705950), located in the promoter region of *MUC5B*, was initially identified in a genetic association study and has been strongly associated with IPF [12]. Several common variants such as *TERT* at 5p15, the 3q26 region near *TERC*, *FAM13A* (4q22), *DSP* (6q24), *OBFC1* (10q24), *ATP11A* (13q34), and *DPP9* (19q13) have been identified [13].

Epidemiological investigations regarding gene–environment interaction affecting the risk of IPF are required.

References

1. Olson AL, Swigris JJ, Lezotte DC, Norris JM, Wilson CG, Brown KK. Mortality from pulmonary fibrosis increased in the United States from 1992 to 2003. Am J Respir Crit Care Med. 2007;176:277–84.
2. Daccord C, Maher TM. Recent advances in understanding idiopathic pulmonary fibrosis. F1000Res 2016;5. pii: F1000 Faculty Rev-1046.
3. Miyake Y, Sasaki S, Yokoyama T, Chida K, Azuma A, Suda T, Kudoh S, Sakamoto N, Okamoto K, Kobashi G, Washio M, Inaba Y, Tanaka H, Japan Idiopathic Pulmonary Fibrosis Study Group. Vegetable, fruit, and cereal intake and risk of idiopathic pulmonary fibrosis in Japan. Ann Nutr Metab. 2004;48:390–7.
4. Miyake Y, Sasaki S, Yokoyama T, Chida K, Azuma A, Suda T, Kudoh S, Sakamoto N, Okamoto K, Kobashi G, Washio M, Inaba Y, Tanaka H. Occupational and environmental factors and idiopathic pulmonary fibrosis in Japan. Ann Occup Hyg. 2005;49:259–65.
5. Miyake Y, Sasaki S, Yokoyama T, Chida K, Azuma A, Suda T, Kudoh S, Sakamoto N, Okamoto K, Kobashi G, Washio M, Inaba Y, Tanaka H, Japan Idiopathic Pulmonary Fibrosis Study Group. Case-control study of medical history and idiopathic pulmonary fibrosis in Japan. Respirology. 2005;10:504–9.
6. Miyake Y, Sasaki S, Yokoyama T, Chida K, Azuma A, Suda T, Kudoh S, Sakamoto N, Okamoto K, Kobashi G, Washio M, Inaba Y, Tanaka H, Japan Idiopathic Pulmonary Fibrosis Study Group. Dietary fat and meat intake and idiopathic pulmonary fibrosis: a case-control study in Japan. Int J Tuberc Lung Dis. 2006;10:333–9.
7. American Thoracic Society. American thoracic society/European Respiratory Society international multidisciplinary consensus classification of the idiopathic interstitial pneumonias. Am J Respir Crit Care Med. 2002;165:277–304.
8. Sasaki S, Yanagibori R, Amano K. Self-administered diet history questionnaire developed for health education: a relative validation of the test-version by comparison with 3-day diet record in women. J Epidemiol. 1998;8:203–15.
9. Sasaki S, Ushio F, Amano K, et al. Serum biomarker-based validation of a self-administered diet history questionnaire for Japanese subjects. J Nutr Sci Vitaminol. 2000;46:285–96.

10. Willett W, Stampfer MJ. Total energy intake: implications for epidemiologic analyses. Am J Epidemiol. 1986;124:17–27.
11. Miyake Y, Fukuoka Heart Study Group. Risk factors for non-fatal acute myocardial infarction in middle-aged and older Japanese. Jpn Circ J. 2000;64:103–9.
12. Seibold MA, Wise AL, Speer MC, Steele MP, Brown KK, Loyd JE, Fingerlin TE, Zhang W, Gudmundsson G, Groshong SD, Evans CM, Garantziotis S, Adler KB, Dickey BF, du Bois RM, Yang IV, Herron A, Kervitsky D, Talbert JL, Markin C, Park J, Crews AL, Slifer SH, Auerbach S, Roy MG, Lin J, Hennessy CE, Schwarz MI, Schwartz DA. A common MUC5B promoter polymorphism and pulmonary fibrosis. N Engl J Med. 2011;364:1503–12.
13. Kaur A, Mathai SK, Schwartz DA. Genetics in idiopathic pulmonary fibrosis pathogenesis, prognosis, and treatment. Front Med (Lausanne). 2017;4:154.

Chapter 8
Epidemiology of Ulcerative Colitis in Japan

Satoko Ohfuji

Abstract In Japan, the prevalence of ulcerative colitis (UC) has been increasing over the past four decades, with the number of patients reaching approximately 170,000 as of 2014. This increase can be partly explained by the broader perception of the disease, improved diagnostic techniques such as endoscopy, and improved disease prognosis resulting from more advanced therapeutic techniques. However, some concerns remain regarding the possibility that a number of environmental factors could be contributing to the increase in the number of UC patients.

To date, numerous studies have been conducted to identify disease risk factors worldwide; however, such studies are faced with the difficulty of showing firm conclusions because of limitations in study designs and statistical power owing to small sample sizes. Therefore, although several factors have been suggested as being associated with UC, the actual burden against disease development remains unclear. Nonetheless, recent improvements in treatment techniques have helped to successfully decrease disease mortality by enabling maintenance of remission in the long-term and prevention of developing colorectal cancers in UC patients.

From a public health perspective, it is important to identify disease risk factors and construct strategies for well-controlling clinical course in UC patients, in order to prevent further new cases and achieve the more improving their prognosis.

Keywords Incidence · Prevalence · Prognosis · Risk factor · Ulcerative colitis

---

S. Ohfuji
Department of Public Health, Osaka City University Graduate School of Medicine, Osaka City, Osaka, Japan
e-mail: satop@med.osaka-cu.ac.jp

M. Washio, G. Kobashi (eds.), *Epidemiological Studies of Specified Rare and Intractable Disease*, Current Topics in Environmental Health and Preventive Medicine, https://doi.org/10.1007/978-981-13-1096-6_8

8.1 Introduction

In Japan in 1975, ulcerative colitis (UC) was officially designated as one of "Nanbyo" (i.e., specified rare intractable diseases) and a subsidy system for medical expenses was launched [1]. UC patients who had specific disease symptoms that matched the disease criteria were then approved to receive aid for their medical expenses by a committee and issued certificates for specific disease treatment. To date, the number of certificates issued for specific disease treatment has increased from 965 in fiscal year 1975, reaching 170,781 throughout Japan as of fiscal year 2014 [1]. This increase can be partly explained by the broader perception of the disease, improved diagnostic techniques such as endoscopy, and improved disease prognosis resulting from more advanced therapeutic techniques. However, some concerns remain regarding the possibility of unknown risk factors contributing to the increase in the number of UC patients.

Here I described the incidence and prevalence of UC from the perspective of descriptive epidemiology, and then focus on the suggested risk and protective factors regarding the development of UC and its prognosis from the perspective of analytic epidemiology.

8.2 Incidence and Prevalence of Ulcerative Colitis

As shown in Table 8.1, the prevalence of UC continues to increase in Japan. In 1984, the prevalence was 7.85 per 100,000 person-years [2]. After sustained increases [3, 4], currently, over 30 years later, the prevalence stands at 134.4 per 100,000 persons [5], which is approximately 20 times higher than that in 1984.

Regarding the incidence and prevalence in the other countries, they are highest in Northern Europe, the United Kingdom (UK), North America, and New Zealand [6]. The incidence and prevalence in these locations have changed dramatically over the past several decades. Research in the USA found the incidence of UC to be 0.6 per 100,000 person-years in the 1940s before surging in the 1970s and reaching 8.3 per 100,000 person-years in the late 1980s, with no substantial increases thereafter. In the early 2000s, UC had a prevalence of 238 per 100,000 persons in the USA and 243 per 100,000 persons in the UK [7]. The figures are two- to sevenfold greater in Western countries than in Japan.

Table 8.1 Incidence and prevalence of ulcerative colitis in Japan

Year	Incidence (per 100,000 person-years)	Prevalence (per 100,000 persons)	References
1984	Not specified	7.85	[2]
1991	1.95	18.1	[3]
2005	Not specified	63.6	[4]
2014	Not specified	134.4	[5]

UC has traditionally been considered to be prevalent in Western countries and unusual in Eastern countries. The incidence, however, began increasing in Japan, as well as in China, South Korea, and India, in the 1980s [6]. An investigation of Indians immigrating to the UK found that first- and second-generation immigrants had a higher incidence of UC than native Indians, and an incidence similar to that of citizens in the UK [8]. Moreover, the incidence of UC was higher in second- than in first-generation immigrants [9]. These findings suggest that Westernized lifestyles and more hygienic environments could contribute to UC onset.

Regarding age distribution, the number of UC patients in Japan peaks among patients in their early 30s, with a second peak in the 50s [4]. This figure is similar to that in Western countries [7]. These observations seem to suggest the possibility that early-onset UC patients are affected by genetic susceptibility, and that late-onset UC patients are affected by a number of lifestyle habits [10].

8.3 Suggested Risk Factors and Preventive Factors for the Development of UC

Between September 2008 and March 2014, we conducted a multicenter case-control study at 38 collaborating hospitals in Japan to investigate risk factors for the development of UC [11]. Newly diagnosed UC patients were recruited as cases, and their lifestyle habits and hygienic environments were compared with those of age- and sex-matched hospital controls. The major results, along with a summary of results from previous studies, are shown in Table 8.2.

In our study [11], the positive association with the development of UC was suggested in patients with family history of inflammatory bowel diseases, past smoker (i.e., quit smoking), higher intake of sweets, peaches or isoflavones, and stressful events, whereas the inverse association was suggested in patients with history of appendicitis, higher intake of particular fruits, and some hygiene factors such as history of acute gastroenteritis and brushing teeth (Table 8.2). In the light of previous studies, I discussed the accumulating results of these suggested factors in the following section.

8.3.1 *Family History of UC*

To date, several studies have consistently indicated that a family history of UC is associated with a higher risk of developing UC [13–20]. Individuals with a family history of UC have been shown to have a 2.3- to 12.5-fold higher risk of developing UC than those without [13–20]. The positive association of family history was reported from not only Japan [11], but also other countries including Greece [13], France [14, 18], Canada [15, 16], China [17], New Zealand [19], and Australia [20].

Table 8.2 Risk factors and preventive factors for the development of ulcerative colitis (UC)

Factor	Finding in our study [11, 12]	Association with the development of UC	References
Family history of inflammatory bowel diseases	OR = 3.33[a]	Positive	[13–20]
History of appendicitis	OR = 0.30[b]	Inverse	[13, 14, 17–31]
Past smoker (quit smoking)	OR = 2.36[b]	Positive	[13, 15–17, 19–21, 23, 32–41]
Current smoker	OR = 0.60	Inverse[c]	
Dietary factors			
Sugars	OR = 0.71	Positive[c]	[21, 33, 38, 42–44]
Japanese sweets	OR = 2.33[b]		
Western sweets	OR = 2.22[b]		
Protein	OR = 0.81	Positive[c]	[15, 44]
Fats, fatty acids	OR = 0.63	Positive[c]	[43, 45]
Fruits	OR = 0.91	Inverse[c]	[21, 38, 42]
Mandarin oranges	OR = 0.51[a]	–	
Strawberries	OR = 0.41[a]	–	
Peaches	OR = 2.05[b]	–	
Vegetables	–	Inverse[c]	[21, 46]
Green/yellow vegs	OR = 0.76	–	
Other vegs	OR = 0.73	–	
Isoflavones	OR = 2.06[b]	–	[12]
Estrogen, oral contraceptives	OR = 1.42	Inverse[c]	[47, 48]
Breast milk	OR = 1.11	Inverse	[19, 21, 32, 37]
Hygiene hypothesis			
Socioeconomic status	OR = 1.32	Inverse[c]/positive[c]	[19]/ [23]
History of acute gastroenteritis	OR = 0.30[b]	Positive[c]	[35, 36]
Oral hygiene (brushing teeth)	OR = 0.55[a]	No association	[38]
Stressful events	OR = 1.69[b]	Positive[c]	[33]

OR odds ratio
[a]$p < 0.1$
[b]$p < 0.05$
[c]Means possible association because of the limited evidences or the inconsistent results

The consistency of the results seemed to indicate the probable association of genetic susceptibility for UC.

All of the previous studies used a case-control study design [11, 13–20], in which only three studies [11, 13, 20] applied incident cases (i.e., newly diagnosed UC patients) as opposed to prevalent cases (i.e., newly diagnosed UC patients and patients who had been diagnosed with UC in the past). However, the studies focusing on family history were not likely to suffer from reverse causality because a family history of UC was considered an inherent characteristic. Thus, even if the results were derived from case-control studies using prevalent cases, their reliability remained high.

Recently, some researches regarding genes related to inflammatory bowel disease have been implementing [16, 49, 50]. I hope to clarify factors determining genetic predisposition and prevent disease onset in the near future.

8.3.2 History of Appendectomy

In our study [11], patients with a history of appendicitis had a significantly decreased risk for developing UC, with odds ratios (ORs) of approximately one-third compared with those without appendicitis history (Table 8.2). Previous Japanese case-control study in 1999–2000 also indicated that patients with appendectomy has about one-third of OR for developing UC [24]. In the other countries, Chinese case-control study also reported that appendectomy was a preventive factor for UC (OR = 0.24) [17]. The inverse association was reported from New Zealand [19] and several European countries including Greece [13], France [14, 18], Denmark [21, 28, 29], the UK [22, 25–27], Spain [23], and Sweden [30].

From the perspective of study design, the inverse association has been reported from not only case-control studies [13, 14, 17–27], but also prospective cohort studies [28–30]. In addition, a meta-analysis concluded that a history of appendectomy was negatively associated with UC onset; the overall OR of appendectomy was 0.307 (95% confidence interval. 0.249–0.377) [31]. Therefore, the inverse association between a history of appendectomy and the development of UC seems to be highly reliable. The risk appears to be particularly low in those who receive an appendectomy before the age of 20 years [22, 28, 30].

Some hypotheses regarding the mechanism underlying this association have been proposed. One hypothesis is that an infection of the appendix might be associated with UC development, because a lower risk has been observed in patients who have had an appendectomy due to appendicitis [22, 28–30]. Another is that an appendectomy may affect the immune system in the colon, because the appendix is an important organ that involves lymphoid tissue that generates IgA-secreting cells to control the composition of microbiota in the colon [51].

8.3.3 Habitual Smoking

Most previous studies have indicated that past smokers (i.e., quit smoking) had higher ORs, whereas current smokers had lower ORs for UC development [13, 15–17, 19–21, 23, 32–41]. Specifically speaking, previous two Japanese case-control studies showed the positive association of past smokers and the inverse association of current smokers for UC [40, 41]. The studies from Australia [20] and New Zealand [19] also suggested these associations, whereas in other Asia-Pacific lesion, one Chinese case-control study reported these associations of smoking habit [17] but another Chinese case-control study failed to show these associations [33].

Besides, a population-based case control study in nine countries of Asia-Pacific revealed that past smokers had an increased OR for UC development but no association of current smokers [32]. In the Western countries, several studies have reported the positive association of past smokers or the inverse association of current smokers from Greece [13], Canada [15, 16], Denmark [21], Spain [23, 34, 35], Sweden/Denmark [36], Italy [37], and the Netherlands [38]. The accumulation of these results has led to the clinical belief that habitual smoking has a protective effect on UC and quit smoking has a harmful effect on UC.

Scrutiny of these studies, however, shows that such findings often originate from case-control studies that used prevalent cases (i.e., newly diagnosed UC patients and patients who have been diagnosed with UC in the past), which may be easily affected by so-called reverse causality [13, 15–17, 19, 23, 36–41]. These studies could be criticized for possibly including UC cases who had quit smoking because of gastrointestinal symptoms prior to diagnosis. If large numbers of such patients were included in UC cases, the observed association between UC and past smokers (i.e., quit smoking) could be biased to be higher, while that between UC and current smokers could be biased to be lower resulting from the reverse causality induced by the study design. To minimize the possibility of reverse causality, the use of incident cases (i.e., newly diagnosed UC patients) has been recommended when conducting case-control studies. To date, the results from case-control studies using incident UC cases have been accumulated [11, 20, 21, 32–35]. These studies similarly found an increased risk of UC onset in past smokers, but the protective effect of current smoking was somewhat obscure in their findings. Therefore, the reported association between current smoking and UC may be apparent because of the reverse causality owing to the study design, although the clinical belief that past smoking (i.e., quit smoking) is a risk factor for the development of UC may be supported.

Why past smoking (i.e., quit smoking) is associated with an increased risk of UC remains unclear. Quit smoking might act as a trigger for the disease onset in a genetically susceptible individual, or might bring about some stresses to the individual, which result in the disease onset. Further studies would be needed to clarify the mechanism of quit smoking for the development of UC.

8.3.4 Dietary Habits

Diet is an important factor because it directly affects the mucosal tissue of the colon. However, there has been limited evidence regarding the association between dietary factors and UC onset. One of the reasons for this lack of evidence is that research on the relationship between diet and UC onset generally faces many challenges, including poor recall of dietary habits and the possibility that participants may unconsciously change their dietary habits before being diagnosed with UC because of its gastrointestinal symptoms. Thus, the results of case-control studies that use prevalent cases are particularly more difficult to interpret.

In our case-control study [11] using incident cases, to consider potential changes in dietary habits owing to disease symptoms, we collected information about the participants' dietary habits during the previous 1 month and 1 year before recruitment. As a result, we found a positive association between a higher consumption of Japanese and Western sweets at 1 year before recruitment and UC onset (Table 8.2). Previous Japanese case-control study also showed the positive association between higher consumption of sweets and the risk of UC [42]. The positive association was also reported from China [33], Israel [43], and European countries such as Denmark [21], the Netherlands [38], and Italy [44]. Although the mechanism is unclear, a higher consumption of sugar might affect the composition of the microbiota in the colon.

Besides, according to previous studies, UC onset could be associated with higher consumption of protein [15, 44] or fats [43, 45]. Although our study failed to detect these associations [11], a Canadian case-control study showed that a high frequency of eating chicken or pork has a higher risk of UC development [15]. A population-based case-control study in Italy supported the result by showing that total protein consumption was significantly higher in UC patients [44]. In addition, a case-control study in Israel indicated that a high fat diet, particularly animal fat and cholesterol, was associated with an increased risk for UC [43]. A case-control study in the Netherlands also reported that high consumption of monounsaturated fat, polyunsaturated fat, and vitamin 6 was associated with an increased risk to develop UC [45].

On the other hand, fruits and vegetables contain antioxidants such as vitamin C, suggesting that a higher consumption of these foods might have a protective effect on UC onset. Although evidence from previous studies is limited [21, 38, 42, 46], our case-control study revealed decreasing ORs in relation to the higher consumption of some fruits such as oranges and strawberries [11]. Previous Japanese case-control study showed the inverse association between high intake of vitamin C and development of UC [42]. A Canadian case control study also indicated that citrus fruit consumption has a decreasing effect for the risk of UC [38]. Regarding the vegetables, a population-based case-control study in Sweden reported that daily intake of vegetables was associated with a decreasing risk of UC [46], and a Danish case-control study also showed that daily intake of fruits and vegetables had a decreasing OR for development of UC [21].

At the present time, however, it is too early to conclude that the abovementioned dietary habits are related to UC onset because very few studies have reported such an association, and no consistent results have been obtained. Further studies are needed to support the relationship between dietary factors and the development of UC.

8.3.5 Effects of Estrogen

Some studies have suggested that oral contraceptives and hormone replacement therapy may increase the risk of UC [47]. A meta-analysis also found that users of an oral contraceptive have a 1.53-fold higher risk of developing UC [48].

Isoflavones have a similar structure to 17b-estradiol; this structural similarity has led some to call the former "dietary estrogen." Our case-control study that investigated the association between isoflavones and UC found that dietary isoflavone consumption was associated with an increased risk of developing UC. This association was pronounced in females, but obscured in males [12]. Therefore, estrogen-mediated pathways might act to promote the development of intestinal inflammation, among females specifically. Further epidemiological and experimental studies including prospective cohort studies are needed to confirm these findings.

8.3.6 Hygiene Hypothesis

According to its descriptive epidemiology, both the incidence and prevalence of UC are higher in Europe and the USA than in other countries. In addition, increasing evidence supports that events early in life may have long-term effects on health and disease. These observations produced the "hygiene hypothesis," which states that exposure to poor hygiene or an increased potential for infection during childhood can confer protection against the development of UC later in life. Although several studies have been conducted to investigate the effect of hygiene on the development of UC [14, 19–21, 23, 25, 27, 32–38], its actual role remains unclear.

In exploring the hygiene hypothesis, various hygiene indicators in childhood have been identified, including breastfeeding, a higher number of siblings, birth order, domestic pets, living place, viral and bacterial infection, vaccination, and sociodemographic factors such as educational level and family income. However, limitations such as poor recall regarding childhood exposure complicate the interpretation of study results. In addition, some hygiene factors are positively associated with UC, whereas others are negatively associated with UC, which makes the role of hygiene on UC development difficult to interpret.

In our case-control study [11], we failed to detect an association between UC and breastfeeding, number of siblings, domestic pets, or family income; however, significantly decreasing ORs were found for history of acute gastroenteritis, and oral hygiene (Table 8.2). A recent animal study indicated that infection with a specific type of *Streptococcus mutans* (i.e., oral bacteria) might confer a risk of UC [52]. Thus, oral hygiene might be important in preventing the development of UC. However, to clearly identify the role of hygiene in relation to the development of UC, more evidence needs to be accumulated in epidemiological and biological studies.

8.4 Prognosis of UC

8.4.1 *Mortality*

According to one study in Japan, among 778 UC patients who had visited eight hospitals from 1973 to 1990, 10-year survival was 96.2%, and no deaths occurred in the 11–18 years after onset [53]. The risk of death was higher in patients with total colitis or in those with acute fulminant colitis. No significant difference was observed in mortality based on age at disease onset (≤29 years, 30–49 years, and ≥ 50 years). Deaths from UC accounted for only about one-sixth of all deaths.

Since treatment modalities, including new medication for UC, have been developing, mortality in the present state might be rapidly improving. Based on a worldwide report from 21 countries, UC mortality showed about a one-fifth decrease from 1951 to 2005, with mortality at 0.12 per 100,000 people in 2000 [54]. Similarly, mortality among UC patients in Japan decreased from 1972 to 2004, and reached 0.10 (men) and 0.07 (women) per 100,000 people in 2004 [55].

Standardized mortality ratios (SMRs) can be used to determine whether mortality among patients with UC is higher than that among the general population, standardized by sex and age. A meta-analysis of mortality among UC patients compared with the general population found that the overall pooled estimate of SMRs was 1.1 (95% confidence interval: 0.9–1.2), suggesting no difference in mortality among UC patients compared with the general population [56]. However, a higher risk of death was reported during the first years of follow-up and in patients with total colitis, where UC-related mortality accounted for 17% of all deaths. Thus, to decrease UC mortality, controlling disease activity in such patients seems to be important.

8.4.2 *Remission and Relapse of Disease Activity*

To improve the long-term prognosis of UC patients, it is important to induce disease activity to the remission state as soon as possible and to maintain the remission state as long as possible. Several treatments have been developed, including 5-aminosalicylic acid products, immunomodulators (azathioprine, 6-mercaptopurine), infliximab infusion, and adalimumab subcutaneous injection, and several studies have investigated their clinical effects in terms of prognosis [57–61].

Table 8.3 summarizes the results of studies in Japan. Remission could be maintained in approximately 60–80% of UC patients within 1 year after medical treatment [57–59]. However, some patients showed a relapse of disease activity during

Table 8.3 Remission and relapse of ulcerative colitis in Japan

Study design/ recruitment period	Study subjects	Follow-up period	Proportion of remission maintenance	Proportion of relapse	Reference
Prospective cohort/2012–2013	4677 patients with 5-aminosalicylic acid products	52 weeks	80.2%	Not specified	[57]
Retrospective cohort/2010–2012	314 patients in remission at 2 weeks after leukocytapheresis	1 year	63.6%	Not specified	[58]
Prospective cohort/2009	99 patients in remission with aminosalicylates	1 year	Not specified	23.1%	[60]
Retrospective cohort/2001–2006	90 patients after leukocytapheresis	Mean 4.6 years	Not specified	69%	[61]

their clinical course [60, 61]. According to the studies from other countries, the proportions of relapse varied in different studies, but were in the ranges of about 30–50% within 1 year, 40% within 2 years, and 60–70% within 5 years after diagnosis [62–68]. However, these proportions were likely affected by age, disease severity, and disease location at the time of diagnosis, as well as adherence or response to treatment, which resulted in the variety seen in the proportion of relapse among the studies.

8.4.3 Onset of Colon Cancer

Patients with UC are widely known to have an increased risk of developing colorectal cancer. A Japanese population-based study reported that an excess mortality from colorectal cancers was observed in the UC patients, especially in males [69]. Western studies have shown that 3.7% of UC patients develop colorectal cancer during their clinical course. The overall incidence was 3/1000 person-years, whereas the risk seemed to be higher in patients with a longer duration of disease. The incidence was 2/1000 person-years during the first decade, 7/1000 during the second, and 12/1000 during the third. The cumulative incidence in patients with UC was 2% by 10 years, 8% by 20, and 18% by 30 [70]. Similar results were also reported in a Japanese study that evaluated the outcomes of 289 UC patients from 1979 to 2014. The cumulative incidence of colorectal cancer was 0.7% by 10 years, 3.2% by 20, 5.2% by 30, and 5.2% by 40, while the cumulative incidence of dysplasia was 3.3% by 10 years, 12.1% by 20, 21.8% by 30, and 29.1% by 40 [71] A meta-analysis, however, showed a decreasing risk of colorectal cancer in UC patients over the past 60 years. The incidence was 4.29/1000 person-years in studies published in the

1950s, but only 1.21/1000 person-years in studies published in the last decade [72]. Improved techniques for medical treatment may have helped to maintain disease remission longer, thereby exerting a positive effect in regard to the prevention of colorectal cancer in UC patients.

8.5 Conclusion

Although the number of UC patients has been increasing in Japan, similar to Western countries, the risk factors underlying disease onset remain largely unknown. Several epidemiological studies have indicated that a combination of genetic and environmental factors affect the risk for developing UC. However, the results of associated studies have not been consistent, and thus a number of suggested factors remain controversial. However, recent improvements in treatment techniques have decreased disease mortality and helped to maintain disease remission in long-term patients and prevent the development of colorectal cancers.

These findings suggest that from a public health perspective, it is important to identify disease risk factors and construct strategies for well-controlling clinical course in UC patients, in order to prevent further new cases and achieve the more improving their prognosis.

References

1. Japan Intractable Diseases Information Center. Number of Recipient Certificates Issued for Specific Disease Treatment (http://www.nanbyou.or.jp/entry/1356) (in Japanese). Accessed 3 Mar, 2018.
2. Higashi A, Watanabe Y, Ozasa K, Hayashi K, Aoike A, Kawai K. Prevalence and mortality of ulcerative colitis and Crohn's disease in Japan. Gastroenterol Jpn. 1988;23:521–6.
3. Morita N, Toki S, Hirohashi T, Minoda T, Ogawa K, Kono S, et al. Incidence and prevalence of inflammatory bowel disease in Japan: nationwide epidemiological survey during the year 1991. J Gastroenterol. 1995;30(Suppl 8):1–4.
4. Asakura K, Nishiwaki Y, Inoue N, Hibi T, Watanabe M, Takebayashi T. Prevalence of ulcerative colitis and Crohn's disease in Japan. J Gasteroenterol. 2009;44:659–65. https://doi.org/10.1007/s00535-009-0057-3.
5. Japanese Ministry of Health, Labour and Welfare. The number of recipient certificates issued for specific disease treatment. 2014. http://www.mhlw.go.jp/toukei/saikin/hw/eisei_houkoku/14/dl/kekka7.pdf. (in Japanese) Accessed 1 Nov 2017.
6. Ananthakrishnan AN. Epidemiology and risk factors for IBD. Nat Rev Gastroenterol Hepatol. 2015;12:205–17. https://doi.org/10.1038/nrgastro.2015.34.
7. Cosnes J, Gower-Rousseau C, Seksik P, Cortot A. Epidemiology and natural history of inflammatory bowel diseases. Gastroenterology. 2011;140:1785–94. https://doi.org/10.1053/j.gastro.2011.01.055.
8. Probert CS, Jayanthi V, Pinder D, Wicks AC, Mayberry JF. Epidemiological study of ulcerative proctocolitis in Indian migrants and the indigenous population of Leicestershire. Gut. 1992;33:687–93.

9. Li X, Sundquist J, Hemminki K, Sundquist K. Risk of inflammatory bowel disease in first- and second- generation immigrants in Sweden: a nationwide follow-up study. Inflamm Bowel Dis. 2011;17:1784–91. https://doi.org/10.1002/ibd.21535.
10. Takahashi H, Matsui T, Hisabe T, Hirai F, Takatsu N, Tsurumi K, et al. Second peak in the distribution of age at onset of ulcerative colitis in relation to smoking cessation. J Gastroenterol Hepatol. 2014;29:1603–8. https://doi.org/10.1111/jgh.12616.
11. Ohfuji S. (2016) Risk factors for inflammatory bowel diseases: A multicenter case-control study. In: Suzuki Y, ed. 2014–2016 Fiscal Year Report of Research Committee on inflammatory bowel diseases (in Japanese). Tokyo: Research on Intractable Diseases, The Ministry of Health, Labour and Welfare of Japan. p. 12–9.
12. Ohfuji S, Fukushima W, Watanabe K, Sasaki S, Yamagami H, Nagahori M, et al. Pre-illness isoflavone consumption and disease risk of ulcerative colitis: a multicenter case-control study in Japan. PLoS One. 2014;9:e110270. https://doi.org/10.1371/journal.pone.0110270.
13. Koutroubakis IE, Vlachonikolis IG, Kapsoritakis A, Spanoudakis S, Roussomoustakaki M, Mouzas IA, et al. Appendectomy, tonsillectomy, and risk of inflammatory bowel disease: case-controlled study in Crete. Dis Colon Rectum. 1999;42:225–30.
14. Baron S, Turck D, Leplat C, Merle V, Gower-Rousseau C, Marti R, et al. Environmental risk factors in paediatric inflammatory bowel diseases: a population based case control study. Gut. 2005;54:357–63.
15. Bernstein CN, Rawsthorne P, Cheang M, Blanchard JF. A population-based case control study of potential risk factors for IBD. Am J Gastroenterol. 2006;101:993–1002.
16. Brant SR, Wang MH, Rawsthorne P, Sargent M, Datta LW, Nouvet F, et al. A population-based case-control study of CARD15 and other risk factors in Crohn's disease and ulcerative colitis. Am J Gastroenterol. 2007;102:313–23.
17. Jiang L, Xia B, Li J, Ye M, Deng C, Ding Y, et al. Risk factors for ulcerative colitis in a Chinese population. An age-matched and sex-matched case-control study. J Clin Gastroenterol. 2007;41:280–4.
18. de Saussure P, Clerson P, Prost PL, Truong Tan N, Bouhnik Y, Gil-Rch. (2007) Appendectomy, smoking habits and the risk of developing ulcerative colitis: a case control study in private practice setting. Gastroenterol Clin Biol 31: 493–497.
19. Gearry RB, Richardson AK, Frampton CM, Dodgshun AJ, Barclay ML. Population-based cases control study of inflammatory bowel disease risk factors. J Gastroenterol Hepatol. 2010;25:325–33. https://doi.org/10.1111/j.1440-1746.2009.06140.x.
20. Abraham N, Selby W, Lazarus R, Solomon M. Is smoking an indirect risk factor for the development of ulcerative colitis? An age- and sex- matched case-control study. J Gastroenterol Hepatol. 2003;18:139–46.
21. Hansen TS, Jess T, Vind I, Elkjaer M, Nielsen MF, Gamborg M, et al. Environmental factors in inflammatory bowel disease: a case-control study based on a Danish inception cohort. J Crohns Colitis. 2011;5:577–84. https://doi.org/10.1016/j.crohns.2011.05.010.
22. Kurina LM, Goldacre MJ, Yeates D, Seagroatt V. Appendicectomy, tonsillectomy, and inflammatory bowel disease: a case-control record linkage study. J Epidemiol Community Health. 2002;56:551–4.
23. López-Serrano P, Pérez-Calle JL, Pérez-Fernández MT, Fernández-Font JM, Boixeda de Miguel D, Fernández-Rodríguez CM. Environmental risk factors in inflammatory bowel diseases. Investigating the hygiene hypothesis: a Spanish case-control study. Scand J Gastroenterol. 2010;45:1464–71. https://doi.org/10.3109/00365521.2010.510575.
24. Naganuma M, Iizuka B, Torii A, Ogihara T, Kawamura Y, Ichinose M, et al. Appendectomy protect against the development of ulcerative colitis and reduces its recurrence: results of a multicenter case-controlled study in Japan. Am J Gastroenterol. 2001;96:1123–6.
25. Duggan AE, Usmani I, Neal KR, Logan RF. Appendicectomy, childhood hygiene, helicobacter pylori status, and risk of inflammatory bowel disease: a case control study. Gut. 1998;43:494–8.
26. Derby LE, Jick H. Appendectomy protects against ulcerative colitis. Epidemiology. 1998;9:205–7.

27. Gent AE, Hellier MD, Grace RH, Swarbrick ET, Coggon D. Inflammatory bowel disease and domestic hygiene in infancy. Lancet. 1994;343:766–7.
28. Frisch M, Pedersen BV, Andersson RE. Appendicitis, mesenteric lymphadenitis, and subsequent risk of ulcerative colitis: cohort studies in Sweden and Denmark. BMJ. 2009;338:b716. https://doi.org/10.1136/bmj.b716.
29. Hallas J, Gaist D, Sørensen HT. Does appendectomy reduce the risk of ulcerative colitis? Epidemiology. 2004;15:173–8.
30. Andersson RE, Olaison G, Tysk C, Ekbom A. Appendectomy and protection against ulcerative colitis. N Engl J Med. 2001;344:808–14.
31. Koutroubakis IE, Vlachonikolis IG. Appendectomy and the development of ulcerative colitis: results of a metaanalysis of published case-control studies. Am J Gastroenterol. 2000;95:171–6.
32. Ng SC, Tang W, Leong RW, Chen M, Ko Y, Studd C, et al. Environmental risk factors in inflammatory bowel disease: a population-based case-control study in Asia-Pacific. Gut. 2015;64:1063–71. https://doi.org/10.1136/gutjnl-2014-307410.
33. Wang YF, Ou-yang Q, Xia B, Liu LN, Gu F, Zhou KF, et al. Mulicenter case-control study of the risk factors for ulcerative colitis in China. World J Gastroenterol. 2013;19:1827–33. https://doi.org/10.3748/wjg.v19.i11.1827.
34. Sicilia B, Arribas F, Nerín J, López Miguel C, Vicente R, Gomollón F. Risk factors for ulcerative colitis: a population-based, case-control study in Spain. J Crohns Colitis. 2008;2:158–61. https://doi.org/10.1016/j.crohns.2008.01.003.
35. García Rodríguez LA, Ruigómez A, Panés J. Acute gastroenteritis is followed by an increased risk of inflammatory bowel disease. Gastroenterol. 2006;130:1588–94.
36. Halfvarson J, Jess T, Magnuson A, Montgomery SM, Orholm M, Tysk C, et al. Environmental factors in inflammatory bowel disease: a co-twin control study of a Swedish-Danish twin population. Inflamm Bowel Dis. 2006;12:925–33.
37. Corrao G, Tragnone A, Caprilli R, Trallori G, Papi C, Andreoli A, et al. Risk of inflammatory bowel disease attributable to smoking, oral contraception and breastfeeding in Italy: a nationwide case-control study. Cooperative investigators of the Italian group for the study of the colon and the rectum (GISC). Int J Epidemiol. 1998;27:397–404.
38. Russel MG, Engels LG, Muris JW, Limonard CB, Volovics A, Brummer RJ, et al. Modern life' in the epidemiology of inflammatory bowel disease: a case-control study with special emphasis on nutritional factors. Eur J Gastroenterol Hepatol. 1998;10:243–9.
39. Fraga XF, Vergara M, Medina C, Casellas F, Bermejo B, Malagelada JR. Effects of smoking on the presentation and clinical course of inflammatory bowel disease. Eur J Gastroenterol Hepatol. 1997;9:683–7.
40. Kurata JH. Dietary and other risk factors of ulcerative colitis. A case-control study in Japan. Epidemiology Group of the Research Committee of inflammatory bowel disease in Japan. J Clin Gastroenterol. 1994;19:166–71.
41. Nakamura Y, Labarthe DR. A case-control study of ulcerative colitis with relation to smoking habits and alcohol consumption in Japan. Am J Epidemiol. 1994;140:902–11.
42. Sakamoto N, Kono S, Wakai K, Fukuda Y, Satomi M, Shimoyama T, et al. Dietary risk factors for inflammatory bowel disease: a multicenter case-control study in Japan. Inflamma Bowel Dis. 2005;11:154–63.
43. Reif S, Klein I, Lubin F, Farbstein M, Hallak A, Gilat T. Pre-illness dietary factors in inflammatory bowel disease. Gut. 1997;40:754–60.
44. Tragnone A, Valpiani D, Miglio F, Elmi G, Bazzocchi G, Pipitone E, et al. Dietary habits as risk factors for inflammatory bowel disease. Eur J Gastroenterol Hepatol. 1995;7:47–51.
45. Geerling BJ, Dagnelie PC, Badart-Smook A, Russel MG, Stockbrügger RW, Brummer RJ. Diet as a risk factor for the development of ulcerative colitis. Am J Gastroenterol. 2000;95:1008–13.
46. Persson PG, Ahlbom A, Hellers G. Diet and inflammatory bowel disease: a case-control study. Epidemiology. 1992;3:47–52.
47. Khalili H, Higuchi LM, Ananthakrishnan AN, Manson JE, Feskanich D, Richter JM, et al. Hormone therapy increases risk of ulcerative colitis but not Crohn's disease. Gastroenterol. 2012;143:1199–206. https://doi.org/10.1053/j.gastro.2012.07.096.

48. Cornish JA, Tan E, Simillis C, Clark SK, Teare J, Tekkis PP. The risk of oral contraceptives in the etiology of inflammatory bowel disease: a meta-analysis. Am J Gastroenterol. 2008;103:2394–400. https://doi.org/10.1111/j.1572-0241.2008.02064.x.
49. Fodil N, Maradin N, Leung V, Olivier JF, Radovanovic I, Jeyakumar T, et al. CCDC88B is required for pathogenesis of inflammatory bowel disease. Nat Commun. 2017;8:932. https://doi.org/10.1038/s41467-017-01381-y.
50. Arisawa T, Nakamura M, Otsuka T, Jing W, Sakurai N, Takano H, et al. Genetic polymorphisms of MAFK, encoding a small Maf protein, are associated with susceptibility to ulcerative colitis in Japan. World J Gastroenterol. 2017;23:5364–70. https://doi.org/10.3748/wjg.v23.i29.5364.
51. Masahata K, Umemoto E, Kayama H, Kotani M, Nakamura S, Kurakawa T, et al. Generation of colonic IgA-secreting cells in the caecal patch. Nat Commun. 2004;5:3704. https://doi.org/10.1038/ncomms4704.
52. Kojima A, Nakano K, Wada K, Takahashi H, Katayama K, Yoneda M, et al. Infection of specific strains of streptococcus mutans, oral bacteria, confers a risk of ulcerative colitis. Sci Rep. 2012;2:332. https://doi.org/10.1038/srep00332.
53. Hiwashita N, Yao T, Watanabe H, Hosoda S, Kobayashi K, Saito T, et al. Long-term follow-up study of ulcerative colitis in Japan. J Gastroenterol. 1995;30(Suppl 8):13–6.
54. Sonnenberg A. Time trends of mortality from Crohn's disease and ulcerative colitis. Int J Epidemiol. 2007;36:890–9.
55. Doi Y, Yokoyama T, Sakai M. Trends in mortality from intractable diseases in Japan, 1972–2004. Nihon Koshu Eisei Zasshi. 2007. 54: 684–94. (in Japanese).
56. Jess T, Gamborg M, Munkholm P, Sørensen TI. Overall and cause-specific mortality in ulcerative colitis: meta-analysis of population-based inception cohort studies. Am J Gastroenterol. 2007;102:609–17.
57. Nagahori M, Kochi S, Hanai H, Yamamoto T, Nakamura S, Omuro S, et al. Real life results in using 5-ASA for maintaining mild to moderate UC patients in Japan, a multi-center study, OPTIMUM study. BMC Gastroenterol. 2009;17:47. https://doi.org/10.1186/s12876-017-0604-y.
58. Kobayashi T, Matsuoka K, Yokoyama Y, Nakamura T, Ino T, Numata T, et al. A multicenter, retrospective, observational study of the clinical outcomes and risk factors for relapse of ulcerative colitis at 1 year after leukocytapheresis. J Gastroenterol. 2018;53:387–96. https://doi.org/10.1007/s00535-017-1356-8.
59. Yokoyama Y, Matsuoka K, Kobayashi T, Sawada K, Fujiyoshi T, Ando T, et al. A large-scale, prospective, observational study of leukocytapheresis for ulcerative colitis: treatment outcomes of 847 patients in clinical practice. J Crohns Colitis. 2014;8:981–91. https://doi.org/10.1016/j.crohns.2014.01.027.
60. Kawakami A, Tanaka M, Nishigaki M, Naganuma M, Iwao Y, Hibi T, et al. Relationship between non-adherence to aminosalicylate medication and the risk of clinical relapse among Japanese patients with ulcerative colitis in clinical remission: prospective cohort study. J Gastroenterol. 2013;48:1006–15. https://doi.org/10.1007/s00535-012-0721-x.
61. Takayama T, Kanai T, Matsuoka K, Okamoto S, Sujino T, Mikami Y, et al. Long-term prognosis of patients with ulcerative colitis treated with cytapheresis therapy. J Crohns Colitis. 2013;7:e49–54. https://doi.org/10.1016/j.crohns.2012.05.005.
62. Romberg-Camps MJ, Dagnelie PC, Kester AD, Hesselink-van de Kruijs MA, Cilissen M, Engels LG, et al. Influence of phenotype at diagnosis and of other potential prognostic factors on the course of inflammatory bowel disease. Am J Gastroenterol. 2009;104:371–83. https://doi.org/10.1038/ajg.2008.38.
63. Leffler D, Cheifetz A. Forecasting the recurrence of ulcerative colitis: can U.C. The future? Inflamm Bowel Dis. 2008;14:422–4.
64. Park SH, Kim YM, Yang SK, Kim SH, Byeon JS, Myung SJ, et al. Clinical features and natural history of ulcerative colitis in Korea. Inflamm Bowel Dis. 2007;13:278–83.
65. Bitton A, Sewitch MJ, Peppercorn MA, deB Edwardes MD, Shah S, Ransil B, et al. Psychosocial determinants of relapse in ulcerative colitis: a longitudinal study. Am J Gastroenterol. 2003;98:2203–8.

66. Kane S, Huo D, Aikens J, Hanauer S. Medication nonadherence and the outcomes of patients with quiescent ulcerative colitis. Am J Med. 2003;114:39–43.
67. Meucci G, Vecchi M, Astegiano M, Beretta L, Cesari P, Dizioli P, et al. The natural history of ulcerative proctitis: a multicenter, retrospective study. Gruppo di studio per le Malattie Infiammatorie Intestinali (GSMII). Am J Gastroenterol. 2000;95:469–73.
68. Moum B, Ekbom A, Vatn MH, Aadland E, Sauar J, Lygren I, et al. Clinical course during the 1st year after diagnosis in ulcerative colitis and Crohn's disease. Results of a large, prospective population-based study in southeastern Norway, 1990-93. Scand J Gastroenterol. 1997;32:1005–12.
69. Ishibashi N, Hirota Y, Ikeda M, Hirohata T. Ulcerative colitis and colorectal cancer: a follow-up study in Fukuoka, Japan. Int J Epidemiol. 1999;28:609–13.
70. Eaden JA, Abrams KR, Mayberry JF. The risk of colorectal cancer in ulcerative colitis: a meta-analysis. Gut. 2001;48:526–35.
71. Kishikawa J, Hata K, Kazama S, Anzai H, Shinagawa T, Murono K, et al. Results of a 36-year surveillance program for ulcerative colitis-associated neoplasia in the Japanese population. Dig Endosc. 2018;30:236–44. https://doi.org/10.1111/den.12955.
72. Castaño-Milla C, Chaparro M, Gisbert JP. Systematic review with meta-analysis: the declining risk of colorectal cancer in ulcerative colitis. Aliment Phartmacol Ther. 2014;39:645–59.

Chapter 9
Epidemiology of Crohn's Disease in Japan

Koji Uchiyama, Mitsumasa Umesawa, Yasuo Haruyama, Toshimi Sairenchi, and Gen Kobashi

Abstract Crohn's disease (CD) is a chronic inflammatory condition of the gastrointestinal tract that most commonly affects the small intestine and colon. Recent data indicate a growing incidence and prevalence of CD worldwide, and CD has become more common in Japan. This report aimed to review the epidemiology of CD in Japan. Japanese genome-wide association studies on CD revealed important race-specific results, such as lack of association with the nucleotide-binding oligomerization domain-containing protein 2 (*NOD2*) locus. Moreover, CD has been considered a multifactorial disease of both genetic and environmental etiology. Therefore, studies on environmental factors and gene–environment interaction analyses are warranted in Japan.

Keywords Crohn's disease · Epidemiological studies · Genetic factors Environmental factors · Westernization · Elemental diets · Pregnancy outcome Japanese

9.1 Introduction

Crohn's disease (CD) is one of main disease phenotypes of inflammatory bowel disease (IBD), often characterized by discontinuous lesions with inflammation that can involve the affected portion of the bowel from the mucosa to the serosa.

K. Uchiyama
Laboratory of International Environmental Health, Center for International Cooperation, Dokkyo Medical University, Tochigi, Japan
e-mail: koji-u@dokkyomed.ac.jp

M. Umesawa · Y. Haruyama · T. Sairenchi · G. Kobashi (✉)
Department of Public Health, Dokkyo Medical University School of Medicine, Tochigi, Japan
e-mail: umesawa@dokkyomed.ac.jp; yasuo-h@dokkyomed.ac.jp; tossair@dokkyomed.ac.jp; genkoba@dokkyomed.ac.jp

M. Washio, G. Kobashi (eds.), *Epidemiological Studies of Specified Rare and Intractable Disease*, Current Topics in Environmental Health and Preventive Medicine, https://doi.org/10.1007/978-981-13-1096-6_9

It mainly affects the small intestine and colon but can involve any portion of the gastrointestinal tract.

Recently, the incidence and prevalence rates of IBD have increased globally, with CD becoming more common in Asian countries with traditionally low incidence, such as Japan, Korea, and China [1]. In Japan, the prevalence rate of CD has more rapidly increased in children than in young adults [2]. This present report aimed to review the recent progress of epidemiological studies on CD in Japan.

9.2 Incidence and Prevalence

The Japanese nationwide CD registry with a public financial aid was launched in 1976, within the framework of measures against intractable diseases compiled in 1972 [3]. Data from the registry, which are accessible to the public, show the number of recipient certificates by age class (in 10-year increments), including recurrence after long-term remission, as shown in Fig. 9.1 [4]. However, additional details are not available. The recently estimated age-standardized registration rate from the registry in 2005–2015 was 1.7 per 100,000 individuals [4], although the recent incidence rates of CD in Japan are unclear. This recent registration rate may

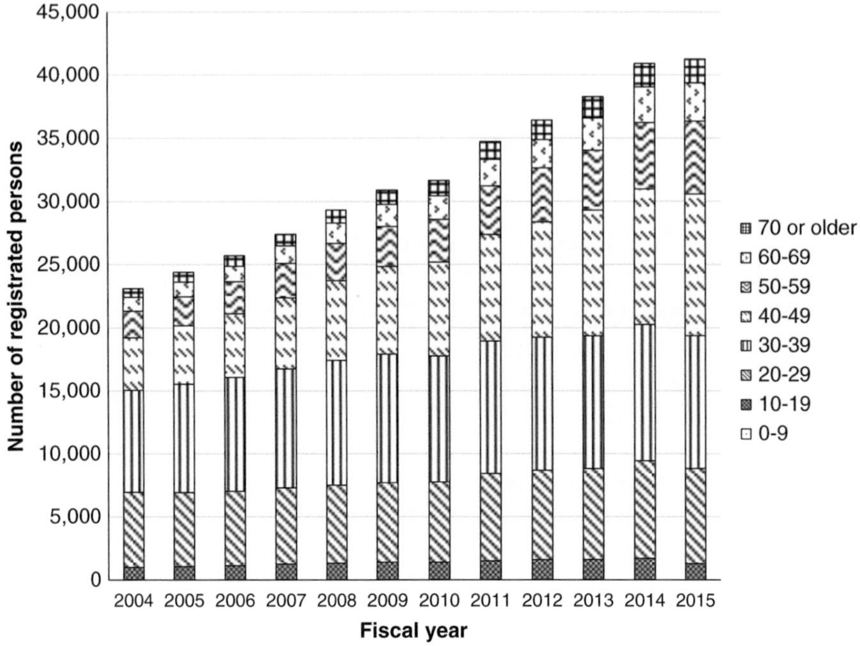

Fig. 9.1 Annual trend of registered CD patients according to age class

indicate that the incidence rates rapidly increased during the last decade, from 0.51 per 100,000 in 1991 [5], as experienced by other Asian countries [1]. In 2015, the Intractable Disease Health Care Act was initiated in Japan [6]. As the act requires a definite diagnosis by designated doctors to register the patient, the characteristics of registrants might have changed before and after 2015. Thus, the recent registration rate may be underestimated. In 2015, a total of 41,279 CD patients were registered, and 1307 (3.2%) were aged ≤19 years. By prefecture, the number of registrants was 3869 (9.4%) in Tokyo, 2986 (7.2%) in Osaka, 2859 (6.9%) in Kanagawa, and 2498 (6.1%) in Aichi. These prefectures were categorized as urban areas in Japan. The order was not changed after adjusting the prefecture's population, making the prevalence rates likely to be higher in urban areas. The prevalence rate increased to 32.5 per 100,000 in 2015, from 30.1 per 100,000 in 2013 [1]. Therefore, the prevalence rate had increased by 8% in just 2 years.

A detailed epidemiological analysis of pediatric IBD using data from the Japanese nationwide registry was performed in 2010 [2]. The study revealed significant differences in sex distribution, family history, and disease severity and extent between adults and children. Men were 1.8 times more likely to have CD than women among adults, compared with 2.6 times higher prevalence in boys than in girls who were ≤16 years in 2005. Among CD children, the proportion of those having a family history of CD was 3.0%; for CD adults, the proportion was 1.7%. Regarding disease severity and extent, the scores at the first registration of pediatric CD, based on the International Organization for the Study of Inflammatory Bowel Diseases, were significantly higher than those of adult CD, and ileum and upper gastrointestinal involvement was observed more commonly in pediatric CD.

9.3 Epidemiology of Clinical Aspects

Another Japanese nationwide database, the Diagnosis Procedure Combination (DPC), was used in a descriptive study of children hospitalized for IBD [7]. Data on 1999 CD and 1560 ulcerative colitis (UC) admissions of 1038 CD and 1137 UC patients aged ≤18 years, who were registered in the DPC database from 2007 to 2010, revealed that 66.4% of admissions were not treated by pediatricians or pediatric surgeons. The admissions included 272 (7.6%) admissions for IBD-related complications, which comprised intestinal (126 admissions of 72 patients), extraintestinal (113 admissions of 88 patients), and other complications (33 admissions of 22 patients). The median duration of hospital stay for CD patients was 6 days (interquartile range [IQR], 2–23 days), shorter than that for UC patients (16 days; IQR, 6–31 days).

In a Japanese cohort study from 1965 to 1998, CD patients with colitis type showed a better clinical course and had significantly different clinical features compared with those with ileitis and ileocolitis types [8].

In a study from medical records of 294 CD patients treated between 1989 and 2009, 13 cancers (6 colorectal, 2 stomach, 2 uterine, 1 small bowel, 1 biliary, and 1 unknown primary site) developed in 12 patients in 4248 person-years [9]. In another study between July 1985 and August 2010, 19 cases of cancer were discovered in 770 CD patients in 10,552 person-years [10].

The reoperation rates after initial surgery in 476 CD patients who were diagnosed between 1963 and 2008 were 31.4% within 5 years and 61.2% within 10 years [11]. It was reported that the onset of CD after 2002, when the antitumor necrosis factor-alpha (TNF-α) antibody drug infliximab was available in Japan, had a protective effect on postoperative recurrence of CD compared with the onset before 2002. Additionally, in the study, postoperative medication of infliximab or immunosuppressant drugs (azathioprine [AZA] and 6-mercaptopurine [6MP]) were risk factors of postoperative recurrence. However, recent studies have reported on the protective effect of the postoperative use of anti-TNF-α antibody drugs, such as the recent introduction of infliximab and adalimumab [12]. The details have not been described, but anti-TNF-α antibody and immunomodulator drugs, when used postoperatively, were reported as protective factors of postoperative recurrence [13]. Moreover, infliximab therapy was associated with improved nutritional status in CD patients [14]. Therefore, the postoperative use of anti-TNF-α drugs may reduce the risk of reoperation; however, further studies are necessary to support such conclusion.

The immunosuppressant drugs AZA and 6MP are thiopurines, which cause serious adverse effects such as leukopenia and hair loss. In a recent study, the homogeneous thymine (T/T) genotype of nudix hydrolase 15 (*NUDT15*) R139C was strongly associated with early (<8 weeks) leukopenia and severe hair loss in Japanese IBD patients [15].

9.4 Genetic Factors

Over the past decade, a meta-analysis of genome-wide association studies (GWASs) has identified over 160 loci associated with IBD in European populations [16]. The loci included not only several IBD general loci, but also some disease phenotype-specific loci.

The nucleotide-binding oligomerization domain-containing protein 2 (*NOD2/CARD15*) locus was one of the CD-specific loci, which was first implicated by linkage analysis [17]. Interestingly, a few studies identified novel *NOD2* mutations, such as P268S mutation in Han Chinese [18] and Zhuang Chinese populations [19] and JW1 and P268S/SNP5 mutations in Malaysian populations [20]. However, significant associations between *NOD2* variants and CD have never been clearly confirmed in Japanese [21] and Korean populations [22]. *NOD2* plays a role in the immune response to intracellular bacterial lipopolysaccharides and subsequently acts as an activator of NF-κB [23]. Therefore, some environmental factors may have ethnic differences through gene–environment interactions.

In 2005, a large-scale case–control study using gene-based single-nucleotide polymorphism (SNP) markers identified that the TNF superfamily member 15 (*TNFSF15*) locus is associated with Japanese CD [24]. *TNFSF15*, which is related to the development of chronic mucosal inflammation by enhancing T-helper type 1 and 17 effector functions [25], was identified as an IBD general locus in European populations [16]. In contrast to *NOD2*, the risk of SNP in *TNFSF15* transcends race, even though an ethnic difference was found in the effect size [26]. Additionally, host–microbiome interaction was proposed as a possible explanation for the ethnic difference in effect size [27].

In 2013, a GWAS compared the genetic characteristics of CD between the European and Japanese populations [28]. In 71 loci, 27 showed at least nominal association, among which 11 remained to show significance even after Bonferroni correction. A meta-analysis of Japanese IBD susceptibility loci was conducted in 2014 [29]. The study identified two CD susceptibility loci in major histocompatibility complex, class II, DR beta 1 (*HLA-DRB1*0405*) and TNF-α (rs1799964 and rs1800630), and two common IBD loci in NK2 transcription factor-related locus 3 (*NKX2-3*, rs10883365) and *TNFSF15* (rs3810936). Recently, a GWAS also compared the genetic characteristics of IBD between the European and Japanese populations [30]. The CD cases were the same as in the previous study [29]; however, a greater number of controls were used. Consequently, five common IBD susceptibility loci, including two East Asian-specific loci, were originally identified. Furthermore, eight CD-specific, four UC-specific, and six common IBD loci from 158 of 163 SNPs reported by European GWASs were confirmed. The results are summarized in Table 9.1.

The human leukocyte antigen (HLA), the major histocompatibility complex in humans, is one of the most polymorphic loci. In a haplotype-based analysis of Japanese GWAS data, distinct effects on CD and UC were reported [31]. The study identified that the *HLA-Cw*1202-B*5201-DRB1*1502* haplotype reduces the risk of CD but increases the risk of UC, which has never been reported in European populations. A few years later, two Japanese CD susceptibility loci, in uncharacterized *LOC105374410* gene (rs1487630) and E74-like ETS transcription factor 1 (*ELF1*, rs7329174), which have never been reported in European CD patients, were identified [32]. These functional and/or ethnic differences between genetic factors and the risk of CD may represent important facets of the etiology of CD.

Generally, the X chromosome is not included in GWASs; meanwhile, as described in Sect. 9.2, significant gender differences were observed in general. As females have two X chromosomes, susceptibility loci for CD on the X chromosome could cause the gender differences. Indeed, Saruta et al. identified both risk (rs4830806) and protective (rs3764879) Toll-like receptor 8 (*TLR8*) haplotypes and clearly showed the association between gender and the risk of American CD through various combinations of these haplotypes [33]. Moreover, an SNP (rs2427870) on the X chromosome was reported as a susceptibility locus in the Korean population [34]. However, no study was ever performed in Japanese CD patients.

Table 9.1 Recently reported IBD susceptibility loci from the Japanese GWAS [30]

Chromosome	Position[a]	SNP	Key genes
East Asian specific (common IBD)			
11	72533536	rs11235604	*ATG16L2*
13	41602462	rs61300271	*ELF1*
CD specific			
2	61204856	rs7608910	*PUS10*
5	72551134	rs7702331	
6	167373547	rs1819333	
9	117553249	rs4246905	*TNFSF15*
10	81032532	rs1250546	*ZMIZ1*
17	57963537	rs1292053	*TUBD1*
19	46849806	rs4802307	*PPP5C*
21	45615741	rs7282490	
IBD shared			
2	27635463	rs1728918	
4	38335067	rs73243351	
5	158826792	rs6871626	
6	32804414	rs241427	*TAP2*
9	117558703	rs6478108	*TNFSF15*
10	35295431	rs11010067	
10	101284237	rs4409764	
14	88472595	rs8005161	*GPR65*
17	40527544	rs12942547	*STAT3*

CD Crohn's disease, *GWAS* genome wide association study, *IBD* inflammatory bowel disease, *SNP* single nucleotide polymorphism

ATG16L2 autophagy related 16 like 2, *ELF1* E74 like ETS transcription factor 1, *GPR65* G-protein coupled receptor 65, *TAP2* transporter 2, adenosine triphosphate binding cassette subfamily B member, *TNFSF15* tumor necrosis factor superfamily member 15, *PPP5C* protein phosphatase 5 catalytic subunit, *PUS10* pseudouridylate synthase 10, *STAT3* signal transducer and activator of transcription 3, *TUBD1* tubulin delta 1, *ZMIZ1* zinc finger MIZ-type containing 1

[a]The position was relative to the NCBI Genome Reference Consortium human build 37 (GRCh37)

9.5 Environmental Factors

Studies on environmental factors in Japan are relatively scarce, although several nutritional investigations, especially regarding CD treatment, have been conducted.

9.5.1 Diet

A high intake of sugars and sweeteners, sweets, fats and oils, and fish and shellfish has been positively associated with an increased risk of CD in Japanese populations [35]. Regarding nutrients, a study also reported that intakes of total fat, monounsaturated and polyunsaturated fatty acids, vitamin E, and n-3 and n-6 fatty acids are positively associated with the risk of CD. According to the European Crohn's and Colitis Organisation's Epidemiological Committee study [36], "Westernization" of lifestyle, such as an increased consumption of refined sugar, fatty acids, and fast food and a reduced consumption of fruits, vegetables, and fibers, might be commonly linked to an increased risk of CD.

To identify food antigens involved in CD, interleukin (IL)-10 knockout (KO) mice experiments and human serological analyses have been performed [37]. One study examined the seroreactivity to immunoglobulin G (IgG) as anti-*Saccharomyces cerevisiae* antibody (ASCA) status was thought to be associated with the risk of CD; indeed, the human serological analyses showed an ASCA IgG-positive rate of 60–70% in CD patients in Western countries [38–41]. In mice experiments, IL-10 KO mice with a C57BL/6 background were used; these mice are well-established animal models for CD [42, 43]. The IL-10 KO mice experiments showed a significant association between food antigens and IgG levels, and the elimination of food antigens improved the IgG levels. However, in a study of 98 Japanese CD patients and 52 Japanese health controls, no significant difference between the number of IgG-positive food items and ASCA IgG levels was found. In contrast, at around the same time, a significant association between the number of positive food antigens and serum IgG values was reported in Chinese CD patients [44]. Typical food items that were significantly associated with increased IgG levels in these studies are summarized in Table 9.2, together with the results of the case–control study in Japan [35] for reference. As can be seen in Table 9.2, no meaningful relationship was found. Meanwhile, a study reported that ASCA positive rates in Japanese CD patients are lower than those in Western CD patients [45]. Recently, food-specific IgG subclasses were found to be not associated with food intolerance and were not altered in German IBD patients [46].

Elemental diets have a relatively long history of use in treating CD worldwide. Elemental diets can be used not only in treating acute CD [47] but also in maintaining remission [48]. After a controlled trial found that using elemental diets in treating acute CD is more effective than using prednisolone [49], elemental diets became one of the established remission-induction therapies for both adult and pediatric CD in Japan [50]. It was also reported that elemental diets reduce mucosal cytokine production, such as IL-1β, IL-1Ra, IL-6, IL-8, and TNF-α, and correct an imbalance between proinflammatory and anti-inflammatory cytokines in CD [51]. In contrast, although exclusive enteral nutrition is the induction therapy of choice for pediatric CD due to its excellent safety profile [52], enteral nutrition for adult CD is not common in other countries, possibly because no significant improvement in efficacy was found, according to a systematic review [53]. However, the role of exclusive enteral nutrition in adult CD is being reexamined [54], and this could be pioneered by the epidemiological studies and clinical experiences in Japan.

A "half-elemental diet" was proposed for the nutritional treatment of CD patients in Japan [55]. This diet can be used as an alternative nutritional maintenance therapy for CD patients who are intolerant or resistant to thiopurines, such as patients with the T/T genotype of *NUDT15* R139C. A half-elemental diet is composed of an elemental diet and usual meals. That is, CD patients take half of their daily allowance

Table 9.2 The relative increasing IgG levels according to food items in CD patients compared with in healthy controls from Japanese and Chinese studies [37, 44], and the odds ratios of CD prevalence according to food items [35]

Food items	IgG level studies		Food items	Case–control study
	Japanese	Chinese		Japanese
Almond	↑	–	Nuts and seeds	→
Lima bean	↑	–		
Peanut	↑	–		
Pecan	↑	–		
Rice	↑	↑	Rice	→
Clam	↑	–	Fish and shellfish	↑
Asparagus	↑	–	Green-yellow vegetables	→
Broccoli	↑	–		
Carrot	↑	–		
Green pepper	↑	–		
Spinach	↑	–		
Tomato	↑	↑		
Cabbage	↑	–	Other vegetables	→
Celery	↑	–		
Cucumber	↑	–		
Lettuce	↑	–		
Onion	↑	–		
Avocado	↑	–	Fruits	→
Grape	↑	–		
Grapefruit	↑	–		
Orange	↑	–		
Mushroom	→	↑	Mushrooms	→
Potato, white	↑	–	Potatoes	→
Beef	→	↑	Meats and poultry	→
Chicken	→	↑		
Egg	→	↑	Eggs	→
Milk	→	↑	Milk and dairy products	→
Yeast	↑	–	Breads	→
Cane sugar	↑	–	Sugars and sweeteners	↑
Buckwheat	↑	–		–
Corn	↑	↑		
Oat	↑	–		
Pinto bean	↑	–		
Soy	↑	↑		
Wheat	→	↑		
Alfalfa	↑	–		
Beets	↑	–		

The symbols "↑" and "→" indicates significantly increased and not found influenced the IgG levels in CD patients (left) or the risk of CD (right), compared to the healthy controls; whereas the symbol "-" means not examined of calories from an elemental diet and take the remaining half from usual unrestricted meals. A randomized trial reported that the recurrence rate of CD in a half-elemental diet group was significantly lower than that in the control group [55]. Moreover, the half-elemental diet was found as effective as the elemental diet in inducing and maintaining remission of CD [56].

9.5.2 Intestinal Microflora

An abnormal response to the gut microbiota is thought to be associated with CD pathogenesis [57]. In several studies performed in Japan [58–61], an increased number of Lactobacillales was commonly observed in Japanese CD patients, whereas no association between *Bacteroides* bacteria and risk of CD occurred. Recently, fecal microbiota transplantation (FMT) has been receiving increased attention as a novel treatment option for IBD. So far, FMT is a safe but variably efficacious treatment for IBD [62]. Thus, FMT could improve the gastrointestinal microbiota ecosystems. However, the mechanisms remain to be elucidated.

9.5.3 Breastfeeding

Breastfeeding was reported to be associated with a lower risk of pediatric CD in Japan [63], as has been believed in Western countries [64]. However, two reports from France in 2005 and Italy in 2017 suggested that breastfeeding is associated with an increased risk of pediatric CD [65, 66]. As the investigation in Japan was conducted from 1979 to 1993 [63], new studies should be carried out to confirm the findings.

9.5.4 Cigarette Smoking

It is well established that active smoking is an independent risk factor of CD [67]. Similarly, it was confirmed that the risk of CD was increased in Japanese smokers [68].

9.6 Pregnancy Outcomes

As described in Sect. 9.2, the onset of CD often occurs during adolescence, affecting individuals during their reproductive years. Thus, CD patients and their families need to know whether disease activity and drug exposures will affect fertility and pregnancy outcomes. A study reported that adverse outcomes such as Caesarean operation and low birth weight were more frequently observed in Japanese women with CD who had a history of surgery for perianal lesions and bowel resection [69]. In another study, exposure to anti-TNF-α treatment or thiopurines during pregnancy was not related to a higher incidence of adverse pregnancy outcomes in Japanese women with IBD without surgery, except for spontaneous abortion [70]. Therefore, further comprehensive studies to reduce such adverse pregnancy outcomes are necessary.

9.7 Summary

An increase in CD prevalence is of concern, and further epidemiological studies are required to reveal the etiology of CD. Despite being the same condition affecting both Western and Japanese populations, CD has been associated with several significant variations in genetic and environmental factors. Hence, more comprehensive epidemiological studies in different races are warranted.

References

1. Ng WK, Wong SH, Ng SC. Changing epidemiological trends of inflammatory bowel disease in Asia. Intest Res. 2016;14:111–9.
2. Ishige T, Tomomasa T, Takebayashi T, Asakura K, Watanabe M, Suzuki T, et al. Inflammatory bowel disease in children: epidemiological analysis of the nationwide IBD registry in Japan. J Gastroenterol. 2010;45:911–7.
3. Ministry of Health, Labour and Welfare: Health and medical services. http://www.mhlw.go.jp/english/wp/wp-hw8/dl/02e.pdf (2014). Accessed 31 Oct 2017.
4. Portal site of official statistics of Japan. http://www.e-stat.go.jp/SG1/estat/NewList.do?tid=000001031469. Accessed 6 Nov 2017.
5. Morita N, Toki S, Hirohashi T, Minoda T, Ogawa K, Kono S, et al. Incidence and prevalence of inflammatory bowel disease in Japan: nationwide epidemiological survey during the year 1991. J Gastroenterol. 1991;30(Suppl 8):1–4.
6. Kanatani Y, Tomita N, Sato Y, Eto A, Omoe H, Mizushima H. National registry of designated intractable diseases in Japan: present status and future prospects. Neurol Med Chir (Tokyo). 2017;57:1–7.
7. Takeuchi M, Tomomasa T, Yasunaga H, Horiguchi H, Fushimi K. Descriptive epidemiology of children hospitalized for inflammatory bowel disease in Japan: inpatient database analysis. Pediatr Int. 2015;57:443–8.
8. Oriuchi T, Hiwatashi N, Kinouchi Y, Takahashi S, Takagi S, Negoro K, et al. Clinical course and longterm prognosis of Japanese patients with Crohn's disease: predictive factors, rates of operation, and mortality. J Gastroenterol. 2003;38:942–53.
9. Mizushima T, Ohno Y, Nakajima K, Kai Y, Iijima H, Sekimoto M, et al. Malignancy in Crohn's disease: incidence and clinical characteristics in Japan. Digestion. 2010;81:265–70.
10. Yano Y, Matsui T, Hirai F, Okado Y, Sato Y, Tsurumi K, et al. Cancer risk in Japanese Crohn's disease patients: investigation of the standardized incidence ratio. J Gastroenterol Hepatol. 2013;28:1300–5.

11. Watanabe T, Sasaki I, Sugita A, Fukushima K, Futami K, Hibi T, et al. Time trend and risk factors for reoperation in Crohn's disease in Japan. Hepato-Gastroenterology. 2012;59:1081–6.
12. Kusaka J, Shiga H, Kuroha M, Kimura T, Kakuta Y, Endo K, et al. Risk factors associated with postoperative recurrence and repeat surgery in Japanese patients with Crohn's disease. Int J Color Dis. 2017;32:1407–13.
13. Shinagawa T, Hata K, Ikeuchi H, Fukushima K, Sugita A, Suzuki Y, et al. Time trends and risk factors for reoperation after initial intestinal surgery for Crohn's disease in Japan: a retrospective multicenter study. Dis Colon Rectum. 2017;60:e412–3.
14. Nakahigashi M, Yamamoto T. Increases in body mass index during infliximab therapy in patients with Crohn's disease: an open label prospective study. Cytokine. 2011;56:531–5.
15. Kakuta Y, Naito T, Onodera M, Kuroha M, Kimura T, Shiga H, et al. NUDT15 R139C causes thiopurine-induced early severe hair loss and leukopenia in Japanese patients with IBD. Pharmacogenomics J. 2016;16:280–5.
16. Jostins L, Ripke S, Weersma RK, Duerr RH, McGovern DP, Hui KY, et al. Host-microbe interactions have shaped the genetic architecture of inflammatory bowel disease. Nature. 2012;491:119–24.
17. Hugot JP, Laurent-Puig P, Gower-Rousseau C, Olson JM, Lee JC, Beaugerie L, et al. Mapping of a susceptibility locus for Crohn's disease on chromosome 16. Nature. 1996;379:821–3.
18. Lv C, Yang X, Zhang Y, Zhao X, Chen Z, Long J, et al. Confirmation of three inflammatory bowel disease susceptibility loci in a Chinese cohort. Int J Color Dis. 2012;27:1465–72.
19. Long WY, Chen L, Zhang CL, Nong RM, Lin MJ, Zhan LL, et al. Association between NOD2/CARD15 gene polymorphisms and Crohn's disease in Chinese Zhuang patients. World J Gastroenterol. 2014;20:4737–44.
20. Chua KH, Hilmi I, Ng CC, Eng TL, Palaniappan S, Lee WS, et al. Identification of NOD2/CARD15 mutations in Malaysian patients with Crohn's disease. J Dig Dis. 2009;10:124–30.
21. Inoue N, Tamura K, Kinouchi Y, Fukuda Y, Takahashi S, Ogura Y, et al. Lack of common NOD2 variants in Japanese patients with Crohn's disease. Gastroenterology. 2002;123:86–91.
22. Croucher PJ, Mascheretti S, Hampe J, Huse K, Frenzel H, Stoll M, et al. Haplotype structure and association to Crohn's disease of CARD15 mutations in two ethnically divergent populations. Eur J Hum Genet. 2003;11:6–16.
23. Pauleau AL, Murray PJ. Role of Nod2 in the response of macrophages to toll-like receptor agonists. Mol Cell Biol. 2003;23:7531–9.
24. Yamazaki K, McGovern D, Ragoussis J, Paolucci M, Butler H, Jewell D, et al. Single nucleotide polymorphisms in TNFSF15 confer susceptibility to Crohn's disease. Hum Mol Genet. 2005;14:3499–506.
25. Takedatsu H, Michelsen KS, Wei B, Landers CJ, Thomas LS, Dhall D, et al. TL1A (TNFSF15) regulates the development of chronic colitis by modulating both T-helper 1 and T-helper 17 activation. Gastroenterology. 2008;135:552–67.
26. Liu JZ, van Sommeren S, Huang H, Ng SC, Alberts R, Takahashi A, et al. Association analyses identify 38 susceptibility loci for inflammatory bowel disease and highlight shared genetic risk across populations. Nat Genet. 2015;47:979–86.
27. Nakagome S, Chinen H, Iraha A, Hokama A, Takeyama Y, Sakisaka S, et al. Confounding effects of microbiome on the susceptibility of TNFSF15 to Crohn's disease in the Ryukyu islands. Hum Genet. 2017;136:387–97.
28. Hirano A, Yamazaki K, Umeno J, Ashikawa K, Aoki M, Matsumoto T, et al. Association study of 71 European Crohn's disease susceptibility loci in a Japanese population. Inflamm Bowel Dis. 2013;19:526–33.
29. Arimura Y, Isshiki H, Onodera K, Nagaishi K, Yamashita K, Sonoda T, et al. Characteristics of Japanese inflammatory bowel disease susceptibility loci. J Gastroenterol. 2014;49:1217–30.
30. Fuyuno Y, Yamazaki K, Takahashi A, Esaki M, Kawaguchi T, Takazoe M, et al. Genetic characteristics of inflammatory bowel disease in a Japanese population. J Gastroenterol. 2016;51:672–81.

31. Okada Y, Yamazaki K, Umeno J, Takahashi A, Kumasaka N, Ashikawa K, et al. HLA-Cw*1202-B*5201-DRB1*1502 haplotype increases risk for ulcerative colitis but reduces risk for Crohn's disease. Gastroenterology. 2011;141:864–71.
32. Yamazaki K, Umeno J, Takahashi A, Hirano A, Johnson TA, Kumasaka N, et al. A genome-wide association study identifies 2 susceptibility loci for Crohn's disease in a Japanese population. Gestroenterology. 2013;144:781–8.
33. Saruta M, Targan SR, Mei L, Ippoliti AF, Taylor KD, Rotter JI. High frequency haplotypes in the X chromosome locus TLR8 are associated with both CD and UC in females. Inflamm Bowel Dis. 2009;15:321–7.
34. Lee HS, Oh H, Yang SK, Baek J, Jung S, Hong M, et al. X chromosome-wide association study identifies a susceptibility locus for inflammatory bowel disease in Koreans. J Crohns Colitis. 2017;11:820–30.
35. Sakamoto N, Kono S, Wakai K, Fukuda Y, Satomi M, Shimoyama T, et al. Dietary risk factors for inflammatory bowel disease: a multicenter case-control study in Japan. Inflamm Bowel Dis. 2005;11:154–63.
36. Burisch J, Pedersen N, Cukovic-Cavka S, Turk N, Kaimakliotis I, Duricova D, et al. Environmental factors in a population-based inception cohort of inflammatory bowel disease patients in Europe – an ECCO-EpiCOM study. J Crohns Colitis. 2014;8:607–16.
37. Kawaguchi T, Mori M, Saito K, Suga Y, Hashioto M, Sako M, et al. Food antigen-induced immune responses in Crohn's disease patients and experimental colitis mice. J Gastroenterol. 2015;50:394–405.
38. Walker LJ, Aldhous MC, Drummond HE, Smith BRK, Nimmo ER, Arnott IDR, et al. Anti-Saccharomyces cerevisiae antibodies (ASCA) in Crohn's disease are associated with disease severity but not NOD2/CARD15 mutations. Clin Exp Immunol. 2004;135:490–6.
39. Quinton JF, Sendid B, Reumaux D, Duthilleul P, Cortot A, Grandbastien B, et al. Anti-Saccharomyces cerevisiae mannan antibodies combined with antineutrophil cytoplasmic autoantibodies in inflammatory bowel disease: prevalence and diagnostic role. Gut. 1998;42:788–91.
40. Peeters M, Joossens S, Vermeire S, Vlietinck R, Bossuyt X, Rutgeerts P. Diagnostic value of anti-saccharomyces cerevisiae and antineutrophil cytoplasmic autoantibodies in inflammatory bowel disease. Am J Gastroenterol. 2001;96:730–4.
41. Ruemmele FM, Targan SR, Levy G, Dubinsky M, Braun J, Seidman EG. Diagnostic accuracy of serological assays in pediatric inflammatory bowel disease. Gastroenterology. 1998;115:822–9.
42. Rennick DM, models FMML f g e a. XII. IL-10-deficient (IL-10$^{-/-}$) mice and intestinal inflammation. Am J Physiol Gastrointest Liver Physiol. 2000;278:G829–33.
43. Hale LP, Greer PK. A novel murine model of inflammatory bowel disease and inflammation-associated colon cancer with ulcerative colitis-like features. PLoS One. 2012;7:e41797.
44. Cai C, Shen J, Zhao D, Qiao Y, Xu A, Jin S, et al. Serological investigation of food specific immunoglobulin G antibodies in patients with inflammatory bowel disease. PLoS One. 2014;9:e112154.
45. Hisabe T, Matsui T, Sakurai T, Murakami Y, Tanabe H, Matake H, et al. Anti-Saccharomyces cerevisiae antibodies in Japanese patients with inflammatory bowel disease: diagnostic accuracy and clinical value. J Gastroenterol. 2003;38:121–6.
46. Jansen A, Mandić AD, Bennek E, Frehn L, Verdier J, Tebrügge I, et al. Anti-food and anti-microbial IgG subclass antibodies in inflammatory bowel disease. Scand J Gastroenterol. 2016;51:1453–61.
47. O'Morain C, Segal AW, Levi AJ. Elemental diets in treatment of acute Crohn's disease. Br Med J. 1980;281:1173–5.
48. Nakahigashi M, Yamamoto T, Sacco R, Hanai H, Kobayashi F. Enteral nutrition for maintainig remission in patients with quiescent Crohn's disease: current status and future perspectives. Int J Color Dis. 2016;31:1–7.

49. Okada M, Yao T, Yamamoto T, Takenaka K, Imamura K, Maeda K, et al. Controlled trial comparing an elemental diet with prednisolone in the treatment of active Crohn's disease. Hepatogastroenterol. 1990;37:72–80.
50. Ueno F, Matsui T, Matsumoto T, Matsuoka K, Watanabe M, Hibi T, et al. Evidence-based clinical practice guidelines for Crohn's disease, integrated with formal consensus of experts in Japan. J Gastroenterol. 2013;48:31–72.
51. Yamamoto T, Nakahigashi M, Umegae S, Kitagawa T, Matsumoto K. Impact of elemental diet on mucosal inflammation in patients with active Crohn's disease: cytokine production and endoscopic and histological findings. Inflamm Bowel Dis. 2005;11:580–8.
52. Ruemmele FM, Veres G, Kolho KL, Griffiths A, Levine A, Escher JC, et al. Consensus guidelines of ECCO/ESPGHAN on the medical management of pediatric Crohn's disease. J Crohns Colitis. 2014;8:1179–207.
53. Zachos M, Tondeur M, Griffiths AM. Enteral nutritional therapy for induction of remission in Crohn's disease. Cochrane Database Syst Rev. 2007;1:CD000542.
54. Wall CL, Day AS, Gearry RB. Use of exclusive enteral nutrition in adults with Crohn's disease: a review. World J Gastroenterol. 2013;19:7652–60.
55. Takagi S, Utsunomiya K, Kuriyama S, Yokoyama H, Takahashi S, Iwabuchi M, et al. Effectiveness of an `half elemental diet` as maintenance therapy for Crohn's disease: a randomized-controlled trial. Aliment Pharmacol Ther. 2006;24:1333–40.
56. Matsui T, Ueki M, Yamada M, Sakurai T, Yao T. Indications and options of nutritional treatment for Crohn's disease. A comparison of elemental and polymeric diets. J Gastroenterol. 1995;30(Suppl 8):95–7.
57. Wright EK, Kamm MA, Teo SM, Inouye M, Wagner J, Kirkwood CD. Recent advances in characterizing the gastrointestinal microbiome in Crohn's disease: a systematic review. Inflamm Bowel Dis. 2015;21:1219–28.
58. Takaishi H, Matsuki T, Nakazawa A, Takada T, Kado S, Asahara T, et al. Imbalance in intestinal microflora constitution could be involved in the pathogenesis of inflammatory bowel disease. Int J Med Microbiol. 2008;298:463–72.
59. Andoh A, Tsujikawa T, Sasaki M, Mitsuyama K, Suzuki Y, Matsui T, et al. Faecal microbiota profile of Crohn's disease determined by terminal restriction fragment length polymorphism analysis. Alient Pharmacol Ther. 2009;29:75–82.
60. Andoh A, Imaeda H, Aomatsu T, Inatomi O, Bamba S, Sasaki M, et al. Comparison of the fecal microbiota profiles between ulcerative colitis and Crohn's disease using terminal restriction fragment length polymorphism analysis. J Gastroenterol. 2011;46:479–86.
61. Fujimoto T, Imaeda H, Takahashi K, Kasumi E, Bamba S, Fujiyama Y, et al. Decreased abundance of Faecalibacterium prausnitzii in the gut microbiota of Crohn's disease. J Gastroenetrol Hepatol. 2013;28:613–9.
62. Colman RJ, Rubin DT. Fecal microbiota transplantation as therapy for inflammatory bowel disease: a systematic review and meta-analysis. J Crohns Colitis. 2014;8:1569–81.
63. Urashima H, Ohmori I, Shiraki K. Epidemiological survey on chronic inflammatory bowel disease developed during childhood in Japan, and a case-control study on nutrition during infancy. Yonago Acta Med. 1999;42:95–102.
64. Klement E, Cohen RV, Boxman J, Joseph A, Reif S. Breastfeeding and risk of inflammatory bowel disease: a systematic review with meta-analysis. Am J Clin Nutr. 2004;80:1342–52.
65. Baron S, Turck D, Leplat C, Merle V, Gower-Rousseau C, Marti R, et al. Environmental risk factors in paediatric inflammatory bowel diseases: a population based case control study. Gut. 2005;54:357–63.
66. Strisciuglio C, Giugliano F, Martinelli M, Genni S, Greco L, Staiano A, et al. Impact of environmental and familial factors in a cohort of pediatric patients with inflammatory bowel disease. J Pediatr Gastroenterol Nutr. 2017;64:569–74.
67. Mahid SS, Minor KS, Soto RE, Hornung CA, Galandiuk S. Smoking and inflammatory bowel disease: a meta-analysis. Mayo Clin Proc. 2006;81:1462–71.

68. Takebayshi T, Nishiwaki Y. Current status of epidemiology of IBD in Japan. In: Hibi T, editor. Recent advances in inflammatory bowel disease. Tokyo: Elsevier; 2007. p. 6–10.
69. Naganuma M, Kunisaki R, Yoshimura N, Nagahori M, Yamamoto H, Kimura H, et al. Conception and pregnancy outcome in women with inflammatory bowel disease: a multicentre study from Japan. J Crohns Colitis. 2011;5:317–23.
70. Komoto S, Motoya S, Nishiwaki Y, Matsui T, Kunisaki R, Matsuoka K, et al. Pregnancy outcome in women with inflammatory bowel disease treated with anti-tumor necrosis factor and/or thiopurine therapy: a multicenter study from Japan. Intest Res. 2016;14:139–45.

Chapter 10
The Role of Gene–Environment Interaction in the Etiology of SLE

Chikako Kiyohara and Masakazu Washio

Abstract Cigarette smoking may be associated with an increased risk of systemic lupus erythematosus (SLE). SLE results from a complex interaction between environmental and genetic risk factors. To evaluate modifying effect of the genetic polymorphisms involved in the metabolism of tobacco smoke on the association of cigarette smoking with SLE risk could be important for understanding of the pathogenesis of SLE. We investigated the relationship of four genetic polymorphisms (cytochrome P450 (*CYP*) *1A1* rs4646903, glutathione S-transferase (*GST*) *M1* deletion and N-acetyltransferase 2 (*NAT2*)) to SLE risk with attention to interaction with cigarette smoking. *CYP1A1* rs4646903 and *NAT2* polymorphisms were significantly associated with SLE risk. The multiplicative interaction between any one of the three genetic polymorphisms and smoking were far from significant. There were significant additive interactions between smoking and either rs4646903 or *NAT2*. Specifically, the attributable proportion due to the interaction was estimated to be approximately 0.50. Future studies involving larger control and case populations, precisely and uniformly defined clinical classification of SLE and better smoking exposure histories will undoubtedly lead to a more thorough understanding of the role of various genes in SLE development.

Keywords Genetic polymorphism · Interaction · SLE · Smoking

C. Kiyohara (✉)
Department of Preventive Medicine, Graduate School of Medical Sciences, Kyushu University, Fukuoka City, Fukuoka, Japan
e-mail: chikako@phealth.med.kyushu-u.ac.jp

M. Washio
Department of Community Health and Clinical Epidemiology, St. Mary's College, Kurume City, Fukuoka, Japan
e-mail: washiomasa@yahoo.co.jp

M. Washio, G. Kobashi (eds.), *Epidemiological Studies of Specified Rare and Intractable Disease*, Current Topics in Environmental Health and Preventive Medicine, https://doi.org/10.1007/978-981-13-1096-6_10

10.1 Introduction

Despite thorough investigation, the etiology of systemic lupus erythematosus (SLE) remains less well-defined. Many environmental exposures, including smoking, alcohol use, ultraviolet light, medications, infectious agents, hair dyes, and dietary factors, have been reported to be associated with the risk of developing SLE [1–5], although the strength of the evidence implicating each of these factors varies. A recent review reported that established environmental risk factors are silica exposure (occupational exposure), Epstein Barr virus exposure, and smoking while less established environmental risk factors are exposures to metals such as mercury, pesticides, halogenated organic compounds, industrial substances, and personal care products [5]. Our studies [6–8] indicated that smoking and alcohol use were possible/probable risk factors for SLE. Smoking has been also suggested to increase the risk of SLE in Western countries [9–12] as well as in Japan [6, 7, 13]. The first meta-analysis of nine epidemiological studies examining this relationship revealed a small but significantly increased risk for the development of SLE among current smokers compared with that among nonsmokers (pooled odds ratio (OR) = 1.50, 95% CI = 1.09–2.08) [3]. The second meta-analysis of 13 epidemiological studies also showed that current smoking increased the risk of SLE (pooled OR = 1.56, 95% CI = 1.26–1.95) [14]. Cigarette smoke affects a wide range of immunological functions in humans [15, 16]. As reactive oxygen species (ROS) promote the autoimmune response [17], exposure to ROS via cigarette smoking may be associated with increased risk of SLE. In contrast to smoking, a meta-analysis reported that no association between moderate alcohol consumption and SLE (summary OR = 0.78, 95% CI = 0.49–1.24) was found when limited to SLE patients treated for less than 5 years while moderate alcohol consumption had a significant protective effect on SLE risk (pooled OR = 0.72, 95% CI = 0.55–0.95) when limited to patients treated for less than 10 years [18]. Ethanol or its metabolites, rather than specific substances in alcoholic beverages, may modulate cytokine release, which in turn will decrease SLE risk [19–23]. The biological mechanisms whereby alcohol may affect SLE remain speculative, however. Taken together, it is plausible that cigarette smoking is associated with SLE risk.

A twin concordance study is commonly used in epidemiology to estimate the role of genetics and the influence of environmental exposures on disease susceptibility. The concordance rate is much higher in monozygotic twins (24–57%) than in dizygotic twins (2–5%), suggesting a genetic contribution to SLE [24, 25]. However, identification of these genetic factors has been slow. The genetic basis of SLE is very complex and it has been estimated that over 100 genes may be involved in the susceptibility to SLE [26].

SLE, like other common multifactorial diseases such as cancers, diabetes, obesity, mental disorder, and cardiovascular disease, results from a complex interaction between environmental and genetic risk factors. However, the disease-provoking factors may include many environmental exposures [27]. In humans, it has been reported that cigarette smoke affects a wide range of immunological functions [15,

16]. In analogy with SLE, rheumatoid arthritis (RA) is autoimmune disease characterized by altered inflammatory and impaired immune responses causing immune-mediated destruction of tissues and organs. In a meta-analysis of 15 studies, current smoking was associated with an increased risk of RA (OR = 1.35 95% CI = 1.17–1.55) [28]. The result of the meta-analysis on RA supports the previous findings that smoking contributes to an increased risk of SLE

It is widely accepted that SLE development requires environmental factors acting on a genetically predisposed individual. Studying gene–environment interactions in relation to SLE risk may be valuable, as positive findings would clearly implicate the substrates with which the gene interacts as disease-causing exposures, clarifying SLE etiology and pointing to environmental modifications for disease prevention. Metabolism of carcinogens related to cigarette smoke is regulated by a balance of a number of steps that involve production and detoxification of ROS. ROS bind covalently to DNA that leads to somatic mutation or disruption of cell cycle. ROS is also considered to promote the autoimmune response [17]. The activities of phase I drug-metabolizing enzymes such as cytochrome P450 (CYP)1A1 and phase II drug-metabolizing (conjugative) enzymes such as S-transferase (GST) M1 are critical for the functionalization of xenobiotics, such as polycyclic aromatic hydrocarbons (PAHs) in cigarette smoke. CYP1A1 contributes to the metabolic activation and formation of ROS, whereas GSTM1 plays a critical role for the detoxification of activated carcinogens or ROS [29, 30]. The enzyme of N-acetyltransferase (NAT) is involved in the metabolism and detoxification of cytotoxic and carcinogenic compounds as well as ROS [31]. It has been suggested that N-acetylation of PAHs by NAT2 may be associated with ROS production [32]. Many researchers have extensively investigated the associations between polymorphisms of *CYP1A1*, *GSTM1,* and *NAT2,* and cancer susceptibility [33–36]. *CYP1A1* rs464903, *GSTM1* deletion, and *NAT2* genotypes determined by *NAT2**4, *5B, *6A, or *7B allele are representative functional polymorphisms. Considering that exposure to cigarette smoking may contribute to the development of SLE, it is important to study the association between SLE and the polymorphisms involved in metabolism of tobacco smoke. In this chapter, we summarized based on our recent studies on interaction between smoking and the genetic polymorphisms involved in metabolism of tobacco smoke in SLE [7, 8, 37, 38].

10.2 Materials and Methods

10.2.1 Study Subjects

The Kyushu Sapporo SLE (KYSS) study was a case–control study to evaluate risk factors for SLE among females [6]. SLE patients (n = 129) were recruited from outpatients of Kyushu University Hospital, Saga University Hospital and their collaborating hospitals in Kyushu from 2002 to 2005, while 51 SLE patients were recruited from outpatients of Sapporo Medical University Hospital and its collaborating hospital in Hokkaido from 2004 to 2005. All patients (n = 180) fulfilled the American College of Rheumatology 1982 revised criteria for SLE [39]. Controls were recruited from nursing college students and care workers in nursing homes in Kyushu (n = 325), while in Hokkaido, controls were recruited from participants at a health clinic (n = 188). Only females who agreed to donate blood samples were included in this study (151 cases and 421 healthy controls). Details of the study subjects have been documented elsewhere [6, 40].

10.2.2 Questionnaire Survey

Cases were asked to complete a self-administered questionnaire about their lifestyles before the diagnosis of SLE while controls completed the questionnaire about their current lifestyles. Subjects were considered current smokers if they smoked or had stopped smoking less than 1 year before either the date of diagnosis (SLE patients) or the date of completion of the questionnaire (controls). The relevant ages would be age at diagnosis (SLE patients) and age at time of questionnaire (controls). Never smokers were defined as those who had never smoked in their lifetime. Former smokers were those who had stopped smoking 1 year or more before either the date of diagnosis (SLE patients) or the date of completion of the questionnaires (controls).

Similarly, subjects were considered current drinkers if they consumed alcohol before either the date of diagnosis of SLE (SLE patients) or completion of the questionnaire (controls). Details of the health examination and the self-administered questionnaire have been documented elsewhere [6, 40].

10.2.3 Genetic Analysis

The *CYP1A1* rs4646903 polymorphism was classified into three genotypes; major genotype (TT), heterozygous genotype (TC), and minor genotype (CC). *GSTM1* genotypes are divided into two categories according to enzymatic activity: null genotype and non-null genotype. The *NAT2* genotypes were classified by this genotyping into three groups: homozygous for the major allele *4/*4 (rapid acetylator), heterozygous for the major and minor alleles *4/*5B, *4/*6A, and *4/*7B (intermediate acetylator), and homozygous for the minor alleles *5B/*5B, *5B/*6A, *5B/*7B, *6A/*6A, *6A/*7B, and *7B/*7B (slow acetylator).

For genotyping quality control, we retyped randomly selected samples (10% of previously typed samples) with the same method and confirmed the complete agreement of genotyping.

10.2.4 Statistical Analysis

Unconditional logistic regression was used to compute the odds ratios (ORs) and their 95% confidence intervals (CIs) with adjustments for several covariates (age, region of residence, smoking status, alcohol consumption). Age was treated as a continuous variable. The remaining covariates were treated as categorical variables. Region of residence fell into two categories (Kyushu and Hokkaido), as did smoking status (current and former smokers combine and never smokers), and alcohol drinking status (current and former drinkers combined and non-drinkers).

The interaction between the genotypes of the four polymorphisms and smoking on the risk of SLE was statistically evaluated based on the likelihood ratio test, comparing the logistic models with and without (multiplicative scale) terms reflecting the product of the genotype and smoking for interaction [41]. In a logistic regression model, interaction refers to a departure from multiplicativity. Rothman has argued that interaction estimated as departure from additivity better reflects biologic interaction [42]. Three measures for biologic interaction as departure from additivity, namely the relative excess risk due to interaction (RERI), attributable proportion (AP), and synergy index (SI) were calculated by the method described by Andersson et al. [43]. Biological interaction was absent if RERI and AP are equal to zero and SI and multiplicative interaction term are equal to one.

All statistical analyses were performed using the computer program STATA Version 12.1 (STATA Corporation, College Station, TX). *p* Values were two-sided, with those less than 0.05 considered statistically significant.

10.3 Results

Table 10.1 shows the association between the polymorphisms involved in the metabolism and detoxification of tobacco smoke and risk of SLE. When adjusted for age, region, smoking status, and alcohol consumption, the CC genotype of *CYP1A1* rs4646903 was significantly associated with an increased risk of SLE (adjusted OR = 2.47, 95% CI = 1.28–4.78) compared with at least one T allele. There was no association between the *GSTM1* deletion polymorphism and SLE risk. As for the *NAT2* acetylator genotypes, the adjusted OR of the intermediate acetylator and slow acetylator genotypes combined was 2.34 (95% CI = 1.36–4.02).

Ever smoking (current and former smokers were combined) was associated with an increased risk of SLE (adjusted OR = 2.86; 95% CI = 1.78–4.60) (data not shown). To achieve adequate statistical power, the genotypes were also categorized into two groups. As significantly higher CYP1A1 enzyme induction was observed

Table 10.1 Association between the polymorphisms involved in the metabolism and detoxification of tobacco smoke and risk of SLE [8, 37]

Genetic polymorphism	Crude OR (95% CI)	Adjusted OR[a] (95% CI)
CYP1A1 rs4646903		
TT genotype	1.00 (reference)	1.00 (reference)
TC genotype	0.96 (0.64–1.43)	0.92 (0.58–1.46)
CC genotype	1.94 (1.07–3.49)	2.37 (1.18–4.78)
CC genotype vs. TT + TC genotypes Combined	1.98 (1.14–3.43)	2.47 (1.28–4.78)
GSTM1 deletion		
Non-null genotype	1.00 (reference)	1.00 (reference)
Null genotype	1.21 (0.84–1.75)	1.13 (0.74–1.73)
NAT2 genotype[b]		
Rapid acetylator genotype	1.00 (reference)	1.00 (reference)
Intermediate acetylator genotype	2.43 (1.46–4.04)	2.18 (1.24–3.85)
Slow acetylator genotype	2.51 (1.41–4.48)	2.34 (1.21–4.52)
Non-rapid[c] genotype vs. rapid Genotype	2.45 (1.50–4.00)	2.34 (1.36–4.02)

CI confidence interval, *OR* odds ratio

[a]Adjusted for age, region, smoking status, and alcohol consumption

[b]Rapid, *4/*4; Intermediate, *4/*5B, *4/*6A, *4/*7B; Slow, *5B/*5B, *5B/*6A, *5B/*7B, *6A/*6A*6A/*7B, *7B/*7B

[c]Intermediate acetylator and slow acetylator genotypes combined

Table 10.2 Interaction between smoking and *CYP1A1* rs4646903 genotypes [8]

		TT + TC genotypes combined		CC genotype	
		Adjusted OR[a] (95% CI)	*p* value	Adjusted OR[a] (95% CI)	*p* value
Smoking status	Never	1.00 (reference)		2.13 (0.98–4.63)	0.055
	Ever	2.73 (1.64–4.54)	<0.0001	9.72 (2.73–34. 6)	<0.0001
			Adjusted OR[a] (95% CI)		*p* value
Multiplicative interaction measure			1.68 (0.37–7.44)		0.503
Additive interaction measure					
Relative excess due to interaction			5.85 (−6.33–18.0)		0.347
Attributable proportion due to interaction			0.60 (0.08–1.13)		0.025
Synergy index			3.04 (0.67–13.9)		0.151

CI confidence interval, *OR* odds ratio

[a]Adjusted for age, region, and alcohol consumption

in subjects with the CC genotype compared with the TT or TC genotype (there was no significant difference in enzymatic activity between the TT genotype and TC genotype) by exposure to smoking [44], the T allele may appear to act in a dominant fashion. The *NAT2* genotypes were classified as rapid acetylator genotype and non-rapid acetylator genotype. Table 10.2 shows the modifying effect of the *CYP1A1* rs4646903 genotypes on the association of smoking with SLE risk. Subjects with the CC genotype (adjusted OR = 9.72, 95% CI = 2.73–34.6) presented a higher risk of SLE than those with at least one T allele (adjusted OR = 2.73, 95% CI = 1.64–4.54) in smokers relative to never smokers with at least one T allele. The multiplicative interaction between the *CYP1A1* rs4646903 genotypes and smoking was not significant. For assessment of additive interaction, adjusted measures (95% CI) of RERI and SI were 5.85 (−6.33–18.0) and 3.04 (0.67–13.9), respectively. These values suggested no significant biologic (additive) interactions. Meanwhile, the adjusted AP due to interaction between the *CYP1A1* rs4646903 genotypes and smoking was estimated to be 0.60 (95% CI = 0.08–1.13; $p = 0.025$), indicating that 60% of the excess risk for SLE in smokers with the CC genotype was due to additive interaction.

Table 10.3 shows the modifying effect of the *GSTM1* genotypes on the association of smoking with SLE risk. Smokers with the *GSTM1* non-null genotype (adjusted OR = 2.32, 95% CI = 1.19–4.52) and smokers with the *GSTM1* null genotype (adjusted OR = 3.35, 95% CI = 1.76–6.39) had a significantly increased risk of SLE. All interaction measures (multiplicative and additive) between the *GSTM1* genotypes and smoking were far from significant, however.

Table 10.4 shows the modifying effect of *NAT2* genotypes on the association of smoking with SLE risk. Individuals with the non-rapid acetylator genotype (adjusted OR = 6.44, 95% CI = 3.07–13.52) presented a higher risk of SLE than those with the rapid acetylator genotype (adjusted OR = 2.16, 95% CI = 0.76–6.15) in smokers, relative to never smokers with the rapid acetylator genotype. The multiplicative interaction between the *NAT2* genotypes and smoking was far from significant. For assessment of additive interaction, adjusted measures (95% CI) of RERI and SI were 3.29 (−0.47–7.05) and 2.40 (0.83–7.00), respectively. These values suggested no significant biologic (additive) interactions. Meanwhile, the adjusted AP due to interaction between the *NAT2* genotypes and smoking was estimated to be 0.50 (95% CI = 0.12–0.88), indicating that 50% of the excess risk for SLE in smokers with the non-rapid acetylator genotype was due to additive interaction.

Table 10.3 Interaction between smoking and *GSTM1* genotypes [8]

		Non-null genotype		Null genotype	
		Adjusted OR[a] (95% CI)	*p* value	Adjusted OR[a] (95% CI)	*p* value
Smoking status	Never	1.00 (reference)		0.98 (0.59–1.65)	0.947
	Ever	2.32 (1.19–4.52)	0.013	3.35 (1.76–6.39)	<0.0001
			Adjusted OR[a] (95% CI)		*p* value
Multiplicative interaction measure			1.47 (0.58–3.69)		0.415
Additive interaction measure					
Relative excess due to interaction			1.04 (−1.17–3.25)		0.356
Attributable proportion due to interaction			0.31 (−0.24–0.86)		0.269
Synergy index			1.79 (0.48–6.69)		0.386

CI confidence interval, *OR* odds ratio

[a]Adjusted for age, region, and alcohol consumption

Table 10.4 Interaction between smoking and *NAT2* genotypes [37]

		Rapid acetylator genotype[a]		Non rapid acetylator genotype[b]	
		Adjusted OR[c] (95% CI)	*p* value	Adjusted OR[c] (95% CI)	*p* value
Smoking status	Never	1.00 (reference)		2.07 (1.07–4.00)	0.055
	Ever	2.16 (0.76–6.15)	0.151	6.44 (3.07–13.52)	<0.0001
			Adjusted OR[c] (95% CI)		*p* value
Multiplicative interaction measure			1.44 (0.45–4.62)		0.536
Additive interaction measure					
Relative excess due to interaction			3.29 (−0.47–7.05)		0.086
Attributable proportion due to interaction			0.50 (0.12–0.88)		0.010
Synergy index			2.40 (0.83–7.00)		0.108

CI confidence interval, *OR* odds ratio
[a]Rapid acetylator genotype, *4/*4
[b]Non-rapid acetylator genotype, intermediate acetylator (*4/*5B, *4/*6A and *4/*7B) and slow acetylator (*5B/*5B, *5B/*6A, *5B/*7B, *6A/*6A, *6A/*7B and *7B/*7B) genotypes combined
[c]Adjusted for age, region, and alcohol consumption

10.4 Discussion

The *CYP1A1* rs4646903, *GSTM1* deletion, and *NAT2* polymorphisms, which are involved in the metabolism and detoxification of tobacco smoke, were genotyped in 151 females with SLE and 421 healthy females in this study. *CYP1A1* rs4646903 and *NAT2* polymorphisms were significantly associated with SLE risk while there was no association between the *GSTM1* deletion polymorphism and SLE risk.

The association between *CYP1A1* polymorphisms and SLE has been reported [45–49]. The *CYP1A1* rs4646903 polymorphism located in the 3′ untranslated region of the *CYP1A1* gene might be involved in the augmented expression of *CYP1A1* mRNA [50]. Moreover, the CC genotype of this polymorphism was associated with increased CYP1A1 inducibility [44]. It is possible that *CYP1A1* rs4646903 is involved in formation of ROS, thereby culminating in inflammation as well as modification of antigens that increases their antigenicity [17]. One Japanese study reported that the *CYP1A1* rs4646903 polymorphism was significantly associated with SLE risk (OR = 1.98, 95% CI = 1.14–3.43) [45] although four studies [46–49] reported no associations.

As enzymatic deficiency in the GSTM1 isoform is correlated with increased risk of certain diseases associated with oxidative damage, it is also possible that there is an association between the *GSTM1* polymorphisms and SLE risk. Glutathione detoxifies ROS, reduces peroxides, and detoxifies multiple compounds through GST conjugation [51, 52]. The *GSTM1* null genotype would be associated with higher ROS. The *GSTM1* null genotype was significantly associated with an increased risk of SLE among Chinese (OR = 1.66, 95% CI = 1.19–2.32) [48] while the recent large GWAS performed in another Chinese population did not detected a significant association [53]. The *GSTM1* null genotype was marginally associated with a decreased risk of SLE among Italian [49]. Other studies found no significant associations [45, 54–57].

As NAT2 is an important xenobiotic-metabolizing enzyme and theoretically the non-acetylated xenobiotics may induce an autoimmune mechanism, the genetic polymorphism of *NAT2* may play a role in susceptibility to SLE. The first study reported a predominance of individuals with slow acetylation activity (slow acetylators) among patients with hydralazine-induced lupus [58]. Furthermore, procainamide-induced lupus appeared to be more common and to develop more rapidly after a smaller cumulative dose in slow acetylators than in rapid acetylators [59]. Hydralazine and procainamide are arylamine drugs. The observation that xenobiotics can cause a drug-induced SLE especially in slow acetylators suggests that non-acetylated xenobiotics may accumulate and convert into reactive metabolites. N-Acetylation is generally accepted as a detoxifying reaction because acetylation indirectly blocks the oxidation of arylamines [60]. Tobacco smoke is a source of the carcinogenic arylamines. Toxic intermediate metabolites of tobacco smoke-derived arylamines are detoxified by NAT2. Therefore, the slow acetylator status is associated with a decreased N-acetylation ability to detoxify toxic compounds, thereby increasing SLE risk. It is hypothesized that these toxic compounds might alter self-proteins presented to the immune system and thus stimulate T-cells which induce pathological and clinical signs of autoimmunity by different effector mechanisms. Furthermore, ROS can be often detoxified by phase II drug-metabolizing enzymes, such as NAT2 [61]. It is plausible that the NAT2 slow acetylator status is associated with an increased risk of SLE. The genetic polymorphism of hepatic NAT2 enzyme causes interindividual variation in response to a variety of amine drugs and potential carcinogens [62, 63]. *NAT2*4* is the major allele. The principal minor alleles that led to a reduction in NAT2 activity are *5B, *6A, and*7B. *NAT2* genotypes are classified as rapid acetylator genotype (two *4 allele (major allele)), intermediate acetylator genotype (one *4 allele), and slow acetylator genotype (no *4 allele). Our previous study found that the *NAT2* slow acetylator status may be a determinant in susceptibility to SLE [37]. The role of the acetylator genotype in the determination of susceptibility to idiopathic SLE is controversial in subsequent studies. Some studies indicated an increased frequency of the slow acetylator phenotype or genotype in SLE patients [46, 64–68], while other studies found no association [69–76]. As ethnic differences in the *NAT2* allele frequencies are striking [63], it has been suggested that the role of the *NAT2* polymorphism on SLE may differ with ethnic group.

Understanding the genetic basis of complex diseases has been increasingly emphasized as a means of achieving insight into disease pathogenesis, with the ultimate goal of improving preventive strategies, diagnostic tools, and therapies. Case–control genetic association studies such as ours aim to detect association between genetic polymorphisms and disease. Although case–control genetic association studies can measure statistical associations, they cannot test causality. Determining genetic causation of disease is a process of inference, which requires supportive results from multiple association studies and basic science experiments combined. Furthermore, a concern with respect to genetic association studies has been lack of replication studies, especially contradictory findings across studies. Additional studies are warranted to replicate our and others' findings from case–control genetic association studies.

It is widely accepted that SLE development requires environmental factors acting on a genetically predisposed individual. Studying gene–environment interactions in relation to SLE risk may be valuable, as positive findings would clearly implicate the substrates with which the gene interacts as disease-causing exposures, clarifying SLE etiology and pointing to environmental modifications for disease prevention. Case–control genetic association study can be useful in investigating gene–environment interactions. Ever smoking was significantly associated with 2.86-fold increased risk of SLE. Substrates for and inducers of CYP1A1 include PAHs such as benzo(a)pyrene in tobacco smoke while GSTM1 detoxifies the metabolites of PAHs. Heterocyclic amines are present in cigarette smoke and are potential substrates for NAT2 activation. Several studies have investigated that smoking was associated with an increased risk of SLE [3]. Cigarette smoking has been proposed to be a trigger for the development of SLE, and the association has been examined in several studies, with conflicting results. Although the biologic pathway through which cigarette smoking acts to increase the instantaneous risk of SLE is not known, several potential mechanisms exist. Exposure to cigarette smoking may be associated with increased risk of SLE. A common method for quantifying interactions is based on the calculation of the two risk factors' product term in a logistic-regression model (multiplicative). A gene–environment interaction was suggested, with "at-risk" genotype and smoking conferring significantly higher risk, compared with no "at-risk" genotype and never smoking in the present study. For example, smokers with "at-risk" genotype of *CYP1A1* rs4646903 was strongly associated with increased risk of SLE (adjusted OR = 9.72, 95% CI = 2.73–34.6). The observed high ORs were attributed largely to the effect of ever-smoking, however. The multiplicative interaction between the genetic polymorphisms and smoking was far from significant, however. Studies of interaction among risk factors in the epidemiological studies have classically been performed using a departure from the additivity model originally described by Rothman, where a term is used to quantify the contribution of interaction to a disease risk, as compared with the contribution of each of the two risk factors added to each other [42, 43]. There were significant additive interactions between smoking and any one of the following: *CYP1A1* rs4646903 or *NAT2* genotypes. Specifically, about 50% of the excess risk for SLE in smokers with the "at-risk" genotype was due to the additive interaction. Thus, the results suggest evidence for additive but not multiplicative interaction. No studies have reported the studies on risk modification by the genetic polymorphisms such as *CYP1A1* rs464903, *GSTM1* deletion, and *NAT2* genotypes determined by *NAT2**4, *5B, *6A, or *7B allele, in the association of cigarette smoking and SLE. Despite the growing awareness of the relevance of gene–environment interactions in human disease, true progress in the identification of common genetic alterations that by themselves may not substantially impact risk, but in concert with environmental exposures may lead to disease development, has been limited. Some genetic variants may exert population-specific effects that are independent of the other genetic profile of the individual and environmental exposures, while other population-specific effects may be generated under differential gene–gene interactions in different populations, differential gene–environment interactions, or both [77]. Sample sizes for adequate power to detect interactions are prohibitively large when the frequencies of interacting variants and exposures are small [77]. In addition, assessment of gene–environment interaction also depends upon the proper statistical evaluation of interaction on the multiplicative and additive models.

Several limitations of this study warrant mention. Our study may have included a bias due to the self-reporting of smoking habits (misclassification bias). However, discrepancies between self-reported smoking habits and biochemical verification are minimal among the general population [78, 79]. Similary, the validity of consumption of coffee and tea using a self-administered questionnaire is relatively high [80, 81]. Recall bias, which occurs when cases and controls recall exposures differently, is also a well-recognized potential problem in case–control studies. SLE patients may be more likely to report their prior exposures than healthy controls because they think they might be related to their disease. The purported link between smoking and SLE is not common knowledge, however. The possibility of recall bias in reporting smoking habit may be minimized, because SLE patients are unlikely to be aware that smoking habit may be associated with SLE risk. Inaccuracies in recall and reporting were possible and, as they were likely nondifferential, could cause dilution of a true association. Population-based case–control studies may have underestimated slightly the true association due to recall bias [82]. Case–control studies tend to be susceptible to selection bias, particularly in the control group. Selection bias may occur if the decision to participate is affected by smoking habit. In many cases, selection bias is not extreme enough to have an impact on inference and conclusions [83]. As the possibility of recall and selection biases could not be completely excluded in case–control studies, our findings should be interpreted with caution. A fundamental conceptual issue selection of controls is whether the controls should be similar to the cases in all respects other than status of the disease in question. As controls were not selected to match SLE patients on confounding factors, there were significant differences between them, such as age. Although matching is one approach to control for confounding bias in the design of the study, the confounding bias can be also controlled for by using statistical modeling approach in the analysis, as was carried out in our study.

In the present study, *CYP1A1* rs4646903 and *NAT2* genotypes were significantly associated with SLE risk. There were significant additive interactions between smoking and any one of the following: *CYP1A1* rs4646903 or *NAT2*. Findings from gene–environment interaction analyses must be interpreted with caution due to reduced numbers of observations in the subgroups. Replication of findings is very important before any causal inference can be drawn. Testing replication in different populations is an important step. Future studies involving larger control and case populations, precisely and uniformly defined clinical classification of SLE and better exposure histories will undoubtedly lead to a more thorough understanding of the role of the genetic polymorphisms involved in the metabolism and detoxification of tobacco smoke in SLE development.

References

1. Montanaro A, Bardana EJ Jr. Dietary amino acid-induced systemic lupus erythematosus. Rheum Dis Clin N Am. 1991;17(2):323–32.
2. Cooper GS, Dooley MA, Treadwell EL, St Clair EW, Parks CG, Gilkeson GS. Hormonal, environmental, and infectious risk factors for developing systemic lupus erythematosus. Arthritis Rheum. 1998;41(10):1714–24. https://doi.org/10.1002/1529-0131(199810)41:10<1714::AID-ART3>3.0.CO;2-U.
3. Costenbader KH, Kim DJ, Peerzada J, Lockman S, Nobles-Knight D, Petri M, et al. Cigarette smoking and the risk of systemic lupus erythematosus: a meta-analysis. Arthritis Rheum. 2004;50(3):849–57. https://doi.org/10.1002/art.20049.
4. Parks CG, Cooper GS. Occupational exposures and risk of systemic lupus erythematosus: a review of the evidence and exposure assessment methods in population- and clinic-based studies. Lupus. 2006;15(11):728–36.
5. Kamen DL. Environmental influences on systemic lupus erythematosus expression. Rheum Dis Clin N Am. 2014;40(3):401–12, vii. https://doi.org/10.1016/j.rdc.2014.05.003.
6. Washio M, Horiuchi T, Kiyohara C, Kodama H, Tada Y, Asami T, et al. Smoking, drinking, sleeping habits, and other lifestyle factors and the risk of systemic lupus erythematosus in Japanese females: findings from the KYSS study. Mod Rheumatol. 2006;16(3):143–50. https://doi.org/10.1007/s10165-006-0474-6.
7. Kiyohara C, Washio M, Horiuchi T, Asami T, Ide S, Atsumi T, et al. Smoking, alcohol consumption, and risk of systemic lupus erythematosus: a case-control study in a Japanese population. J Rheumatol. 2012;39(7):1363–70. https://doi.org/10.3899/jrheum.111609.
8. Kiyohara C, Washio M, Horiuchi T, Asami T, Ide S, Atsumi T, et al. Risk modification by CYP1A1 and GSTM1 polymorphisms in the association of cigarette smoking and systemic lupus erythematosus in a Japanese population. Scand J Rheumatol. 2012;41(2):103–9. https://doi.org/10.3109/03009742.2011.608194.
9. Hardy CJ, Palmer BP, Muir KR, Sutton AJ, Powell RJ. Smoking history, alcohol consumption, and systemic lupus erythematosus: a case-control study. Ann Rheum Dis. 1998;57(8):451–5.
10. Ghaussy NO, Sibbitt WL Jr, Qualls CR. Cigarette smoking, alcohol consumption, and the risk of systemic lupus erythematosus: a case-control study. J Rheumatol. 2001;28(11):2449–53.
11. Formica MK, Palmer JR, Rosenberg L, McAlindon TE. Smoking, alcohol consumption, and risk of systemic lupus erythematosus in the black women's health study. J Rheumatol. 2003;30(6):1222–6, [pii]: 0315162X-30-1222
12. Ekblom-Kullberg S, Kautiainen H, Alha P, Leirisalo-Repo M, Julkunen H. Smoking and the risk of systemic lupus erythematosus. Clin Rheumatol. 2003;32(8):1219–22. https://doi.org/10.1007/s10067-013-2224-4.
13. Nagata C, Fujita S, Iwata H, Kurosawa Y, Kobayashi K, Kobayashi M, et al. Systemic lupus erythematosus: a case-control epidemiologic study in Japan. Int J Dermatol. 1995;34(5):333–7.
14. Jiang F, Li S, Jia C. Smoking and the risk of systemic lupus erythematosus: an updated systematic review and cumulative meta-analysis. Clin Rheumatol. 2015;34(11):1885–92. https://doi.org/10.1007/s10067-015-3008-9.
15. Sopori ML, Kozak W. Immunomodulatory effects of cigarette smoke. J Neuroimmunol. 1998;83(1–2):148–56.
16. Hersey P, Prendergast D, Edwards A. Effects of cigarette smoking on the immune system. Follow-up studies in normal subjects after cessation of smoking. Med J Aust. 1983;2(9):425–9.
17. Griffiths HR. Is the generation of neo-antigenic determinants by free radicals central to the development of autoimmune rheumatoid disease? Autoimmun Rev. 2008;7(7):544–9. https://doi.org/10.1016/j.autrev.2008.04.013.
18. Wang J, Pan HF, Ye DQ, Su H, Li XP. Moderate alcohol drinking might be protective for systemic lupus erythematosus: a systematic review and meta-analysis. Clin Rheumatol. 2008;27(12):1557–63. https://doi.org/10.1007/s10067-008-1004-z.

19. Imhof A, Froehlich M, Brenner H, Boeing H, Pepys MB, Koenig W. Effect of alcohol consumption on systemic markers of inflammation. Lancet. 2001;357(9258):763–7. https://doi.org/10.1016/S0140-6736(00)04170-2, [pii]: S0140-6736(00)04170-2
20. Ripley BJ, Goncalves B, Isenberg DA, Latchman DS, Rahman A. Raised levels of interleukin 6 in systemic lupus erythematosus correlate with anaemia. Ann Rheum Dis. 2005;64(6):849–53. https://doi.org/10.1136/ard.2004.022681, [pii]: 64/6/849
21. McCarty MF. Interleukin-6 as a central mediator of cardiovascular risk associated with chronic inflammation, smoking, diabetes, and visceral obesity: down-regulation with essential fatty acids, ethanol and pentoxifylline. Med Hypotheses. 1999;52(5):465–77. https://doi.org/10.1054/mehy.1997.0684, [pii]: S0306-9877(97)90684-8
22. Wirleitner B, Schroecksnadel K, Winkler C, Schennach H, Fuchs D. Resveratrol suppresses interferon-gamma-induced biochemical pathways in human peripheral blood mononuclear cells in vitro. Immunol Lett. 2005;100(2):159–63. https://doi.org/10.1016/j.imlet.2005.03.008, [pii]: S0165-2478(05)00069-6
23. Cho KH, Kim HJ, Rodriguez-Iturbe B, Vaziri ND. Niacin ameliorates oxidative stress, inflammation, proteinuria, and hypertension in rats with chronic renal failure. Am J Physiol Renal Physiol. 2009;297(1):F106–13. https://doi.org/10.1152/ajprenal.00126.2009, [pii]: 00126.2009
24. Jarvinen P, Aho K. Twin studies in rheumatic diseases. Semin Arthritis Rheum. 1994;24(1):19–28, [pii]: 0049-0172(94)90096-5
25. Deapen D, Escalante A, Weinrib L, Horwitz D, Bachman B, Roy-Burman P, et al. A revised estimate of twin concordance in systemic lupus erythematosus. Arthritis Rheum. 1992;35(3):311–8.
26. Tsao BP. Update on human systemic lupus erythematosus genetics. Curr Opin Rheumatol. 2004;16(5):513–21, [pii]: 00002281-200409000-00005
27. David SP. Systemic lupus erythematosus B. Epidemiology, pathology, and pathogenesis. In: Klippel JH, Stone JH, Crofford LJ, White PH, editors. Primer on the rheumatic diseases. 13th ed. New York: Springer-Verlag; 2008. p. 319–26.
28. Sugiyama D, Nishimura K, Tamaki K, Tsuji G, Nakazawa T, Morinobu A, et al. Impact of smoking as a risk factor for developing rheumatoid arthritis: a meta-analysis of observational studies. Ann Rheum Dis. 2010;69(1):70–81. https://doi.org/10.1136/ard.2008.096487.
29. Nebert DW, Dalton TP. The role of cytochrome P450 enzymes in endogenous signalling pathways and environmental carcinogenesis. Nat Rev Cancer. 2006;6(12):947–60. https://doi.org/10.1038/nrc2015, [pii]: nrc2015
30. Hayes JD, Flanagan JU, Jowsey IR. Glutathione transferases. Annu Rev Pharmacol Toxicol. 2005;45:51–88. https://doi.org/10.1146/annurev.pharmtox.45.120403.095857.
31. Unal M, Tamer L, Dogruer ZN, Yildirim H, Vayisoglu Y, Camdeviren H. N-acetyltransferase 2 gene polymorphism and presbycusis. Laryngoscope. 2005;115(12):2238–41. https://doi.org/10.1097/01.mlg.0000183694.10583.12.
32. Kim WJ, Lee HL, Lee SC, Kim YT, Kim H. Polymorphisms of N-acetyltransferase 2, glutathione S-transferase mu and theta genes as risk factors of bladder cancer in relation to asthma and tuberculosis. J Urol. 2000;164(1):209–13.
33. Masson LF, Sharp L, Cotton SC, Little J. Cytochrome P-450 1A1 gene polymorphisms and risk of breast cancer: a HuGE review. Am J Epidemiol. 2005;161(10):901–15. https://doi.org/10.1093/aje/kwi121.
34. Castelao JE, Yuan JM, Skipper PL, Tannenbaum SR, Gago-Dominguez M, Crowder JS, et al. Gender- and smoking-related bladder cancer risk. J Natl Cancer Inst. 2001;93(7):538–45.
35. Parl FF. Glutathione S-transferase genotypes and cancer risk. Cancer Lett. 2005;221(2):123–9. https://doi.org/10.1016/j.canlet.2004.06.016.
36. Agundez JA. Polymorphisms of human N-acetyltransferases and cancer risk. Curr Drug Metab. 2008;9(6):520–31.
37. Kiyohara C, Washio M, Horiuchi T, Tada Y, Asami T, Ide S, et al. Cigarette smoking, N-acetyltransferase 2 polymorphisms and systemic lupus erythematosus in a Japanese population. Lupus. 2009;18(7):630–8. https://doi.org/10.1177/0961203309102809.

38. Kiyohara C, Washio M, Horiuchi T, Asami T, Ide S, Atsumi T, et al. The modifying effect of NAT2 genotype on the association between systemic lupus erythematosus and consumption of alcohol and caffeine-rich beverages. Arthritis Care Res. 2014;66:1048. https://doi.org/10.1002/acr.22282.
39. Tan EM, Cohen AS, Fries JF, Masi AT, McShane DJ, Rothfield NF, et al. The 1982 revised criteria for the classification of systemic lupus erythematosus. Arthritis Rheum. 1982;25(11):1271–7.
40. Kiyohara C, Washio M, Horiuchi T, Takahashi H, Tada Y, Kobashi G, et al. Dietary patterns and the risk of systemic lupus erythematosus in a Japanese population: the Kyushu Sapporo SLE (KYSS) study. Int Med J. 2015;22(3):110–5.
41. Marshall SW. Power for tests of interaction: effect of raising the type I error rate. Epidemiol Perspect Innov. 2007;4:4. https://doi.org/10.1186/1742-5573-4-4.
42. Rothman KJ. Measuring interaction. Epidemiology: an introduction. New York: Oxford University Press; 2002. p. 168–80.
43. Andersson T, Alfredsson L, Kallberg H, Zdravkovic S, Ahlbom A. Calculating measures of biological interaction. Eur J Epidemiol. 2005;20(7):575–9.
44. Kiyohara C, Hirohata T, Inutsuka S. The relationship between aryl hydrocarbon hydroxylase and polymorphisms of the CYP1A1 gene. Jpn J Cancer Res. 1996;87(1):18–24, [pii]:0910505096845650
45. Horiuchi T, Washio M, Kiyohara C, Tsukamoto H, Tada Y, Asami T, et al. Combination of TNF-RII, CYP1A1 and GSTM1 polymorphisms and the risk of Japanese SLE: findings from the KYSS study. Rheumatology (Oxford). 2009;48(9):1045–9. https://doi.org/10.1093/rheumatology/kep166.
46. von Schmiedeberg S, Fritsche E, Ronnau AC, Specker C, Golka K, Richter-Hintz D, et al. Polymorphisms of the xenobiotic-metabolizing enzymes CYP1A1 and NAT-2 in systemic sclerosis and lupus erythematosus. Adv Exp Med Biol. 1999;455:147–52.
47. Yen JH, Chen CJ, Tsai WC, Lin CH, Ou TT, Hu CJ, et al. Manganese superoxide dismutase and cytochrome P450 1A1 genes polymorphisms in rheumatoid arthritis in Taiwan. Hum Immunol. 2003;64(3):366–73. https://doi.org/S0198885902008182, [pii]
48. Zhang J, Deng J, Zhang C, Lu Y, Liu L, Wu Q, et al. Association of GSTT1, GSTM1 and CYP1A1 polymorphisms with susceptibility to systemic lupus erythematosus in the Chinese population. Clin Chim Acta. 2010;411(11-12):878–81. https://doi.org/10.1016/j.cca.2010.03.007, [pii]: S0009-8981(10)00176-2
49. Rupasree Y, Naushad SM, Rajasekhar L, Kutala VK. Association of genetic variants of xenobiotic metabolic pathway with systemic lupus erythematosus. Indian J Biochem Biophys. 2013;50(5):447–52.
50. Landi MT, Bertazzi PA, Shields PG, Clark G, Lucier GW, Garte SJ, et al. Association between CYP1A1 genotype, mRNA expression and enzymatic activity in humans. Pharmacogenetics. 1994;4(5):242–6.
51. Hayes JD, Strange RC. Glutathione S-transferase polymorphisms and their biological consequences. Pharmacology. 2000;61(3):154–66, [pii]: pha61154
52. Landi S. Mammalian class theta GST and differential susceptibility to carcinogens: a review. Mutat Res. 2000;463(3):247–83, [pii]: S1383574200000508
53. Han JW, Zheng HF, Cui Y, Sun LD, Ye DQ, Hu Z, et al. Genome-wide association study in a Chinese Han population identifies nine new susceptibility loci for systemic lupus erythematosus. Nat Genet. 2009;41(11):1234–7. https://doi.org/10.1038/ng.472, [pii]: ng.472
54. Ollier W, Davies E, Snowden N, Alldersea J, Fryer A, Jones P, et al. Association of homozygosity for glutathione-S-transferase GSTM1 null alleles with the Ro+/La- autoantibody profile in patients with systemic lupus erythematosus. Arthritis Rheum. 1996;39(10):1763–4.
55. Tew MB, Ahn CW, Friedman AW, Reveille JD, Tan FK, Alarcon GS, et al. Systemic lupus erythematosus in three ethnic groups. VIII. Lack of association of glutathione S-transferase null alleles with disease manifestations. Arthritis Rheum. 2001;44(4):981–3. https://doi.org/10.1002/1529-0131(200104)44:4<981::AID-ANR158>3.0.CO;2-0.
56. Fraser PA, Ding WZ, Mohseni M, Treadwell EL, Dooley MA, St Clair EW, et al. Glutathione S-transferase M null homozygosity and risk of systemic lupus erythematosus associated

with sun exposure: a possible gene-environment interaction for autoimmunity. J Rheumatol. 2003;30(2):276–82, [pii]: 0315162X-30-276
57. Kang TY, El-Sohemy A, Comelis MC, Eny KM, Bae SC. Glutathione S-transferase genotype and risk of systemic lupus erythematosus in Koreans. Lupus. 2005;14(5):381–4.
58. Perry HM Jr, Tan EM, Carmody S, Sakamoto A. Relationship of acetyl transferase activity to antinuclear antibodies and toxic symptoms in hypertensive patients treated with hydralazine. J Lab Clin Med. 1970;76(1):114–25.
59. Woosley RL, Drayer DE, Reidenberg MM, Nies AS, Carr K, Oates JA. Effect of acetylator phenotype on the rate at which procainamide induces antinuclear antibodies and the lupus syndrome. N Engl J Med. 1978;298(21):1157–9. https://doi.org/10.1056/nejm197805252982101.
60. Hein DW. Acetylator genotype and arylamine-induced carcinogenesis. Biochim Biophys Acta. 1988;948(1):37–66.
61. Jana S, Mandlekar S. Role of phase II drug metabolizing enzymes in cancer chemoprevention. Curr Drug Metab. 2009;10(6):595–616.
62. Evans D. N-acetyltransferases. In: Kalow W, editor. Pharmacogenetics of drug metabolism. New York: Pergamon Press; 1992. p. 95–197.
63. Hein DW, Doll MA, Fretland AJ, Leff MA, Webb SJ, Xiao GH, et al. Molecular genetics and epidemiology of the NAT1 and NAT2 acetylation polymorphisms. Cancer Epidemiol Biomark Prev. 2000;9(1):29–42.
64. Foad B, Litwin A, Zimmer H, Hess EV. Acetylator phenotype in systemic lupus erythematosus. Arthritis Rheum. 1977;20(3):815–8.
65. Larsson R, Karlsson E, Molin L. Spontaneous systemic lupus erythematosus and acelylator phenotype. Acta Med Scand. 1977;201(3):223–6.
66. Fishbein E, Alarcon-Segovia D. Slow acetylation phenotype in systemic lupus erythematosus. Arthritis Rheum. 1979;22(1):95–7.
67. Johansson E, Mustakallio KK, Mattila MJ. Polymorphic acetylator phenotype and systemic lupus erythematosus. Acta Med Scand. 1981;210(3):193–6.
68. Reidenberg MM, Martin JH. The acetylator phenotype of patients with systemic lupus erythematosus. Drug Metab Dispos. 1974;2(1):71–3.
69. Sardas S, Karakaya AE, Sardas OS. Acetylator phenotype in patients with systemic lupus erythematosus. Arthritis Rheum. 1986;29(11):1412–3.
70. Kumana CR, Chan MM, Wong KL, Wong RW, Kou M, Lauder IJ. Lack of association between slow acetylator status and spontaneous lupus erythematosus. Clin Pharmacol Ther. 1990;48(2):208–13.
71. Ong ML, Mant TG, Veerapen K, Fitzgerald D, Wang F, Manivasagar M, et al. The lack of relationship between acetylator phenotype and idiopathic systemic lupus erythematosus in a South-east Asian population: a study of Indians, Malays and Malaysian Chinese. Br J Rheumatol. 1990;29(6):462–4.
72. Shiokawa S, Yasuda M, Nobunaga M. Genotypes of polymorphic arylamine N-acetyltransferase in systemic lupus erythematosus. Arthritis Rheum. 1992;35(11):1397–9.
73. Reidenberg MM, Drayer DE, Lorenzo B, Strom BL, West SL, Snyder ES, et al. Acetylation phenotypes and environmental chemical exposure of people with idiopathic systemic lupus erythematosus. Arthritis Rheum. 1993;36(7):971–3.
74. Zschieschang P, Hiepe F, Gromnica-Ihle E, Roots I, Cascorbi I. Lack of association between arylamine N-acetyltransferase 2 (NAT2) polymorphism and systemic lupus erythematosus. Pharmacogenetics. 2002;12(7):559–63.
75. Cooper GS, Treadwell EL, Dooley MA, St Clair EW, Gilkeson GS, Taylor JA. N-acetyl transferase genotypes in relation to risk of developing systemic lupus erythematosus. J Rheumatol. 2004;31(1):76–80.
76. Rychlik-Sych M, Skretkowicz J, Gawronska-Szklarz B, Gornik W, Sysa-Jedrzejowska A, Skretkowicz-Szarmach K. Acetylation genotype and phenotype in patients with systemic lupus erythematosus. Pharmacol Rep. 2006;58(1):22–9.
77. Hunter DJ. Gene-environment interactions in human diseases. Nat Rev Genet. 2005;6(4):287–98. https://doi.org/10.1038/nrg1578, [pii]: nrg1578

78. Patrick DL, Cheadle A, Thompson DC, Diehr P, Koepsell T, Kinne S. The validity of self-reported smoking: a review and meta-analysis. Am J Public Health. 1994;84(7):1086–93.
79. Wells AJ, English PB, Posner SF, Wagenknecht LE, Perez-Stable EJ. Misclassification rates for current smokers misclassified as nonsmokers. Am J Public Health. 1998;88(10):1503–9.
80. Mannisto S, Virtanen M, Mikkonen T, Pietinen P. Reproducibility and validity of a food frequency questionnaire in a case-control study on breast cancer. J Clin Epidemiol. 1996;49(4):401–9.
81. Ferraroni M, Tavani A, Decarli A, Franceschi S, Parpinel M, Negri E, et al. Reproducibility and validity of coffee and tea consumption in Italy. Eur J Clin Nutr. 2004;58(4):674–80. https://doi.org/10.1038/sj.ejcn.1601864.
82. Giovannucci E, Stampfer MJ, Colditz GA, Manson JE, Rosner BA, Longnecker MP, et al. Recall and selection bias in reporting past alcohol consumption among breast cancer cases. Cancer Causes Control. 1993;4(5):441–8.
83. Geneletti S, Richardson S, Best N. Adjusting for selection bias in retrospective, case-control studies. Biostatistics. 2009;10(1):17–31. https://doi.org/10.1093/biostatistics/kxn010.

Chapter 11
Epidemiological Studies of Specified Rare and Intractable Disease

TNF Receptor-Associated Periodic Syndrome (TRAPS)

Naoyasu Ueda and Takahiko Horiuchi

Abstract Tumor necrosis factor receptor-associated periodic syndrome (TRAPS) is a representative of autoinflammatory diseases. We conducted a nationwide survey for patients with *TNFRSF1A* variants in Japan. We obtained clinical and genetic features of 51 patients from 33 independent families. The most common variant was T61I (appearing in 49% of patients), and it was identified in 7 of 363 healthy controls. The common clinical features of Japanese patients were fever of >38 °C (100% of patients), arthralgia (59%), and rash (55%). The prevalence of abdominal pain (36%), myalgia (43%), and amyloidosis (0%) was significantly lower in Japanese patients than in Caucasian patients. Patients with *TNFRSF1A* variants are very rare in Japan, as in other countries, but there are a number of clinical and genetic differences between Japanese and Caucasian patients.

Keywords Tumor necrosis factor receptor-associated periodic syndrome (TRAPS) · *TNFRSF1A* · Japan · Japanese · T61I

11.1 Introduction

Tumor necrosis factor receptor-associated periodic syndrome (TRAPS) is a representative of autoinflammatory diseases. It is a rare disease, and has been reported mainly in Caucasians [1]. However, as reports in Japanese also increased, the Ministry of Health, Labor, and Welfare (MHLW) of Japan organized a study group for TRAPS chaired by Professor Horiuchi of Kyushu University. A nationwide survey revealed that there are at least 33 families of TRAPS in Japan [2]. In this

N. Ueda
Department of Internal Medicine, Miyazaki Prefectural Miyazaki Hospital, Miyazaki, Japan

T. Horiuchi (✉)
Department of Internal Medicine, Kyushu University Beppu Hospital, Beppu, Japan
e-mail: horiuchi@beppu.kyushu-u.ac.jp

M. Washio, G. Kobashi (eds.), *Epidemiological Studies of Specified Rare and Intractable Disease*, Current Topics in Environmental Health and Preventive Medicine, https://doi.org/10.1007/978-981-13-1096-6_11

chapter, we first describe the disease concept and pathophysiology of TRAPS. Next, the results of the nationwide survey and characteristics of TRAPS in Japan which the nationwide survey revealed are described. TRAPS has been certified as "Nanbyo" (intractable disease) on January 1, 2015.

11.2 Disease Concept

TRAPS is an autosomal dominant inherited autoinflammatory disease caused by mutations of the TNF receptor super family 1A (*TNFRSF1A*) gene encoding type 1 TNF receptor (TNFR1). Representative diseases of autoinflammatory diseases involve familial Mediterranean fever (FMF), mevalonate kinase deficiency (MKD), cryopyrin-associated periodic syndrome (CAPS) in addition to TRAPS, each of which is characterized by recurrent inflammatory episodes with fever and various organ involvements. The term autoinflammation was made to denote a group of diseases without the usual features of autoimmunity (high-titer autoantibodies and autoreactive T cells), which were subsequently recognized as disorders of the innate immune system [3]. TRAPS was originally reported as familial perireticular amyloidosis, familial Hibernian fever (FHF), and autosomal dominant familial periodic syndrome. In 1998, genome-wide association study revealed that both disease susceptibility loci of FHF and autosomal dominant familial periodic syndrome are located on chromosome 12p3 [4, 5]. In 1999, mutations in the *TNFRSF1A* gene were identified and led to the naming of TRAPS [6]. TRAPS is characterized clinically by recurrent inflammatory episodes such as fever, myalgia, joint pain, rash, periorbital edema, conjunctivitis, and serositis. Severe cases complicate amyloidosis. Although it often occurs in childhood, adult onset cases are also seen [1].

11.3 Pathophysiology

TNFR1 is a transmembrane protein consisting of 455 amino acid (Fig. 11.1). The extracellular domain of TNFR1 consists of four cysteine-rich domains (CRD1-4), each of which contains three cysteine–cysteine disulfide bonds [7]. CRD1, also known as the pre-ligand assembly domain (PLAD), mediates self-assembly in the absence of ligand [8]. The ligand binding domains are made up of CRD2 and CRD3. The intracellular region includes a death domain (DD) that can initiate signaling cascades for both inflammation and apoptosis. Soluble TNFR1, corresponding to TNFR1 extracellular domain, is shed by proteolytic cleavage. The major TNFR1 cleavage site is in the spacer region adjacent to the transmembrane domain between Asn-172 and Val-173, with a minor site between Lys-174 and Gly-175 [9]. *TNFRSF1A* consists of 10 exons. For example, the latter half of exon 2 and the first half of exon 3 encode CRD1. Figure 11.1 shows the location of *TNFRSF1A* variants. *TNFRSF1A* variants seen in TRAPS patients are concentrated in exon 2, 3, and

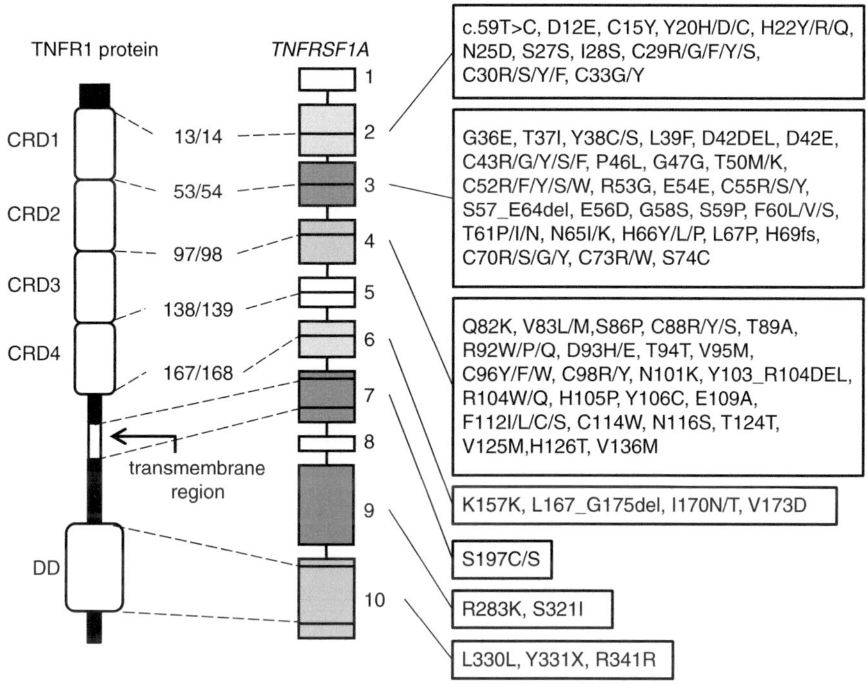

Fig. 11.1 Schematic representations of TNFR1 protein, *TNFRSF1A* gene and *TNFRSF1A* sequence variants. TNFR1 is a transmembrane protein consisting of 455 amino acid. The extracellular domain of TNFR1 consists of four cysteine-rich domains (CRD1–4). The intracellular region includes a death domain (DD). The *TNFRSF1A* gene consists of 10 exons. The locations of *TNFRSF1A* variants are shown. The numbering of the amino acids for *TNFRSF1A* has not followed the general rule of starting with the translation initiator methionine, as most publications have started numbering after the leading sequence, i.e., leucine at residue 30

4 encoding CRD1, CRD2, and CRD3. The numbering of the amino acids for *TNFRSF1A* has not followed the general rule of starting with the translation initiator methionine, as most publications have started numbering after the leading sequence, i.e., leucine at residue 30. Also in this chapter numbering is done as such. The list of variants of the genes responsible for autoinflammatory diseases, including TRAPS, is maintained and updated in the Infevers database (http://fmf.igh.cnrs.fr/infevers).

Currently, the leading hypothesis of pathological mechanisms of TRAPS is the defect of intracellular trafficking of mutated TNFR1 [10, 11]. The *TNFRSF1A* mutation causes misfolding of the TNFR1 protein structure. The misfolding TNFR1 is not transported to the secretory pathway after the Golgi apparatus by the protein quality control mechanism, resulting in intracellular retention of mutated TNFR1 in the endoplasmic reticulum (ER). Because of autophagic abnormality, mutated TNFR1 is not degraded, and accumulates in the ER [12]. Accumulation of mutated TNFR1 enhances the production of reactive oxygen species (ROS) from mitochondria. Mitochondrial ROS activates mitogen-activated protein kinase (MAPK) through suppression of MAPK dephosphorylation [13]. Accumulation of mutated

TNFR1 causes ER stress response and increases expression of ER stress-related proteins such as Spliced X-box binding protein 1 (sXBP1). sXBP1 enhances inflammatory cytokine production induced by Toll-like receptor (TLR) stimulation in ROS dependence [14]. By these mechanisms, inflammatory cytokine production such as TNF-α, IL-6, and pro-IL-1β is induced against a small amount of lipopolysaccharide (LPS) stimulation that normally does not react.

The *TNFRSF1A* mutations causing functional abnormalities such as intracellular trafficking defect in TNFR1 are referred to as "structural mutations" [11]. Representatives of "structural mutations" are mutations of cysteine residues that form disulfide bonds and the T50M mutation which is a mutation of threonine residue that form hydrogen bonds that are presumed to have a major influence on the structure of TNFR1. *TNFRSF1A* mutations such as defects in cysteine residues and the T50M mutation have not been found in patients other than TRAPS patients and asymptomatic patient relatives, whereas the R92Q and P46L variants are found in allele frequencies of about 1% in the Caucasian general population. The R92Q and P46L variants are associated with low penetrance and a mild TRAPS phenotype. A few patients with R92Q and P46L develop amyloidosis [15]. Functional abnormalities such as intracellular trafficking defect are not observed in the R92Q and P46L TNFR1. The R92Q and P46L variants are referred to as "nonstructural" [11].

It is a matter of debate whether the P46L and R92Q variants really have a pathogenic effect. In West African individuals without TRAPS-like symptoms, the allele frequency of the P46L variant is as high as 9.8% [16]. The allele frequency of the R92Q variant in children with periodic fever (2.45%) did not differ significantly from the allele frequency in healthy subjects (2.25%) in Italy [17]. It has been suggested that the R92Q variant might be a susceptibility factor in other inflammatory diseases. The frequency of the R92Q variant tended to be higher in patients with early arthritis, but this finding is a subject of controversy [18, 19]. The R92Q variant was also significantly more frequent in patients with Behçet's disease, atherosclerosis, and idiopathic recurrent endocarditis than in healthy controls [20–22]. Genome-wide association studies identified the R92Q variant as a genetic risk factor for multiple sclerosis [23].

11.4 Diagnosis

TRAPS is diagnosed by genetic testing. Hull and colleagues have proposed "Diagnostic indicators of TRAPS" composed of items including symptoms and family history [1]. It should be noted that this is not a diagnostic criteria but a guideline for judging the indication of genetic testing. It is difficult to diagnose TRAPS only by clinical findings. Clinical findings such as age of onset, clinical symptoms, frequency and duration of inflammatory attack, severity of disease, and therapeutic response vary considerably among patients [24]. There is a possibility of TRAPS even in cases where symptoms such as myalgia and abdominal pain are main symptoms and fever is not observed or patients in whom disease course is continuous rather than periodic (recurrent). Atypical case was reported who was completely asymptomatic until the development of amyloidosis [25]. Additionally, the *TNFRSF1A* variants are often not identified in patients who are clinically consistent as TRAPS. It was reported that *TNFRSF1A* variants were identified in 10 families among 18 families in which multiple members had symptoms compatible with TRAPS and only 4 of 176 subjects with sporadic TRAPS-like symptoms [26]. In patients with recurrent inflammatory episodes, if etiologies such as infections, neoplasms, and other rheumatic conditions are unlikely, genetic testing of *TNFRSF1A* should be considered.

11.5 Treatment

If inflammatory attack is mild and infrequent, you can treat only symptomatic relief with NSAIDs alone. Colchicine and immunosuppressive agents such as methotrexate and cyclosporin are considered ineffective [1].

The most common therapeutic agents are corticosteroids. After terminating the attack using high dose corticosteroids, you should promptly taper and discontinue corticosteroids. In some cases, it is difficult to taper and discontinue corticosteroids because the required amount increases during the course or severe attacks occur frequently. Corticosteroid complications such as osteoporosis are a major problem in cases requiring high doses and long-term corticosteroid administration. For such cases the use of biological agents should be considered [27, 28].

Currently, IL-1 inhibition is a first-line biological agent. A phase-II clinical study demonstrated clear efficacy for canakinumab, leading to US Food and Drug Administration (FDA) approval of the drug for the treatment of TRAPS [29]. Also in Japan, canakinumab received approval for the treatment of TRAPS in December 2016.

Etanercept, one of TNF inhibitors, can be effective in some patients. However, the response is partial and loss of efficacy occurs in most cases [30]. The use of infliximab and adalimumab, which are TNF inhibitors, are associated with exacerbation of TRAPS and should be avoided [31–33]. Etanercept is a type 2 TNF receptor-Fc fusion protein, while infliximab and adalimumab are a monoclonal antibody. This structural difference may cause a difference in clinical effect.

11.6 Epidemiological Findings of TRAPS Before Our National Survey

From Germany, an epidemiological national survey of pediatric patients was reported in 2009 [34]. Monthly inquiries were sent to 370 children's hospitals and pediatric rheumatological outpatient clinics and to all 23 laboratories performing genetic analyses for Hereditary periodic fever. In July 2003 to June 2006, they found 23 new patients. The incidence of TRAPS in German children was estimated to be ~5.6 per 10^7 person-years, and it was concluded that TRAPS is a rare disease in Caucasians. 19 (83%) of 23 cases had the R92Q variant, which is a variant of uncertain pathogenic significance. If we consider only *TNFRSF1A* mutations with clearly pathogenic significance, the incidence is even lower.

Case series of 158 patients was reported in 2013 from the Eurofever/EUROTRAPS international registry, which is a web-based registry collected retrospective data on patients with *TNFRSF1A* sequence variants and inflammatory symptoms [24]. The median age at which symptoms began was 4.3 years but 9.1% of patients presented after 30 years of age. The most common *TNFRSF1A* variant was R92Q (34% of cases), followed by T50M (10%). Defect of cysteine residues were found in 27% of cases. A family history was present in 19% of patients with R92Q and 64% of those with other variants.

The first confirmed case of TRAPS in Japan was a female patient with the C70S mutation and was reported in 2003 [35]. She was also the first case in an eastern Asian population. Before our national survey, the number of Japanese patient with genetically confirmed TRAPS were 18 patients from 9 independent families [36]. A national survey for FMF was conducted twice in 2006 and 2009 and this revealed that a significant number of patients with FMF exist in Japan and Japanese FMF patients were clinically or genetically different from Mediterranean patients [37, 38]. With these backgrounds, our national survey was conducted.

11.7 Primary Survey

The MHLW study group for TRAPS conducted a national survey. In 2010, we mailed a questionnaire to all 1718 internal medicine departments and 1182 pediatric departments in hospitals with more than 200 beds, asking whether they had patients in whom TRAPS was suspected from January to December 2009. Contacting hospitals with more than 200 beds was determined to be enough to find patients with undiagnosed TRAPS, because it was presumed that patients with undiagnosed TRAPS are referred to large hospitals as patients with recurrent fever of unknown cause. The criteria for TRAPS were not set and were left up to each doctor's judgment in order to widely screen patients in whom TRAPS was suspected. However, to assist physicians with finding TRAPS patients, we advised recruiting into the study patients who either (1) fulfilled Hull's classification criteria for TRAPS [1] or (2) presented atypical symptoms of juvenile idiopathic arthritis (JIA) or adult-onset Still's disease (AOSD). "Atypical disease" was defined as disease without chronic arthritis or with recurrent inflammatory attacks. It is noteworthy that a number of TRAPS patients were misdiagnosed as having atypical systemic JIA [39]. A total of 826 of 1718 internal medicine departments (48.1%) and 981 of 1182 pediatrics departments (83.0%) responded to our questionnaire (Table 11.1). There were 263 patients in whom TRAPS was clinically suspected. The number of patients in whom TRAPS was clinically suspected nationwide was estimated in units of institutions,

Table 11.1 Results of mailed questionnaire survey to 2900 departments in the hospitals with more than 200 beds

		No. of departments	Response rate (n)	%	No. of departments reporting Suspected TRAPS patients	No. of reported patients	Estimated patient number
Internal medicine	University hospitals	97	63	64.9	16	32	49.3
	≥500 beds	304	155	50.9	18	42	82.4
	400–499 beds	239	131	54.8	13	24	43.8
	300–399 beds	490	216	44.3	16	33	74.9
	200–299 beds	588	261	44.3	11	13	29.3
	Total	1718	826	48	74	144	279.6
Pediatrics	University hospitals	97	76	80.8	21	35	43.3
	≥500 beds	262	212	80.9	16	24	29.7
	400–499 beds	197	181	91.8	13	18	19.6
	300–399 beds	335	291	86.8	19	27	31.1
	200–299 beds	294	221	75.1	11	15	20
	Total	1182	961	82.9	80	119	143.6
Total		2900	1807	62.3	154	263	423.2

assuming that there was a random response regardless of the number of patients. That is, we weighted by the reciprocal of the response rate and estimated the total number of patients by Stata version 11 (Stata Coop., Texas USA). As a result, it was estimated that there were 423 patients in whom TRAPS was clinically suspected nationwide.

11.8 Secondary Survey

We then asked the departments that replied that they had patients in whom TRAPS was clinically suspected to provide detailed clinical information and a blood sample for genetic testing. A total of 169 patients underwent genetic analysis in our study. Genetic testing of a total of 359 healthy controls was also conducted. All individuals were Japanese. The study was approved by the ethics committee of Kyushu University. Written informed consent was obtained from each enrolled patient. Screening for mutations of all the coding exons of the *TNFRSF1A* (exons 1–10),

MEFV (exons 1–10), and *MVK* (exons 2–11) genes was performed by direct sequencing. *TNFRSF1A* variants were identified in 10 patients from 10 independent families. The T61I variant was found in 8 patients, while the V136M and S321I variants were found in 1 patient each. All the patients were heterozygous for the variants. Among the healthy controls, 7 of 363 individuals were heterozygous for the T61I variant. There was no significant difference in the allele frequency of the T61I variant between the patient group and the control group; however, there was a trend toward an increased frequency of the T61I variant in the patient group ($p = 0.071$). *TNFRSF1A* variants other than the T61I variant were not identified in healthy individuals. The R92Q and P46L variants, which are associated with low penetrance and a mild TRAPS phenotype and are present in about 1% of the Caucasian general population, were not observed in our patients or controls.

Although *MEFV* variants/polymorphisms were found in many patients and healthy individuals, mutations in exon 10, which are considered most pathogenic, were found in only 2 of the 159 patients without any *TNFRSF1A* variants. One patient was heterozygous for the Y688C *MEFV* mutation, but the patient was clinically diagnosed as having AOSD. The other was heterozygous for the M694I *MEFV* mutation and satisfied the Tel Hashomer criteria for FMF [40]. Therefore, this patient was diagnosed as having FMF. Heterozygous V109 L and D386N *MVK* variants were found in 1 patient each. One healthy individual was carrying the V109L variant. The 2 patients with these *MVK* variants were not carrying any *TNFRSF1A* variants. As MKD is an autosomal-recessive inherited disease, the MVK mutation needs to be homozygous to cause the disease. Therefore, the pathogenic role of these 2 variants is not clear.

In this study, we found 10 patients with *TNFRSF1A* variants, from 10 independent families. In addition, we collected information on 17 patients from 13 independent families with *TNFRSF1A* variants and symptoms of inflammation who had not been described in the literature. A total of 27 patients from 23 families were shown in Table 11.2. The C15Y, V125 M, V136 M, and S321I variants were novel variants found in this study. A literature search revealed that 24 additional cases from 11 families with *TNFRSF1A* variants and symptoms of inflammation had been reported from Japan [35, 39, 41–48]. In total, clinical and genetic features of 51 patients from 33 independent families were obtained (Table 11.3).

11.9 Genetic Features of Patients with TNFRSF1A Variant in Japan

Defects in cysteine residues and the T50M variant referred to as "structural mutations" were found in 33% of the 51 patients with *TNFRSF1A* variant. T61I was the most common variant, found in 19 families, followed by the C30Y and T50M variants in two families each. The sporadic cases included 14 patients with the T61I variant and 1 patient each with the C15Y, N101K, V136M, and S321I variants. Among the sporadic cases, the parents of five patients with the T61I variant and the

Table 11.2 Characteristics of 27 patients with *TNFRSF1A* variants in Japan newly identified in this study

Family	Case	*TNFRSF1A* variant	Variants in other genes	Family history	Gender	Age at onset, years	Duration of episode, days	Fever (>38 °C)	Abdominal pain	Myalgia	Skin rash	Conjunctivitis	Periorbital edema	Chest pain	Arthralgia	Headache	Amyloidosis	CRP during attack (mg/dl)	CRP between attacks (mg/dl)	Other observations	Response to NSAID	Response to corticosteroid	Respond to etanercept	Respond to colchicine
1	1	C15Y	ND	–	M	9	7–14	+	+	+	–	–	–	–	+	+	–	7.1	0.1		–	+	++	–
2	2	T50 M	ND	+	M	1	5–21	+	+	–	+	+	–	–	+	+	–	8.1	ND		ND	++	ND	ND
3	3	C70S[a]	–	+	F	20	7-14	+	–	+	+	–	+	–	–	–	–	ND	ND		+	NA	NA	NA
4	4	T61I	E148Q in *MEFV*; Q49K in *PSMB8*	–	M	53	Continuous	+	–	–	+	–	–	+	+	–	–	17.2	ND	Pericarditis	ND	++	NA	NA
5	5	T61I	R471C in *NOD2*; Q49K in *PSMB8*	–	F	12	10–16	+	–	+	+	+	–	–	+	–	–	17.6	0.2		++	NA	NA	NA
6	6	T61I	E148Q in *MEFV*; G39V in *NLRP12*; Q49K in *PSMB8*	–	F	0.5	7–21	+	–	+	+	+	+	+	+	+	–	ND	0.0	Her sister is homozygous for T61 but asymptomatic.	–	++	NA	NA
7	7	T61I	E148Q in *MEFV*; Q49K in *PSMB8*	–	M	65	1	+	–	–	–	–	–	–	–	–	–	7.8	4.5		–	NA	NA	NA

(continued)

Table 11.2 (continued)

Family	Case	*TNFRSF1A* variant	Variants in other genes	Family history	Gender	Age at onset, years	Duration of episode, days	Fever (>38 °C)	Abdominal pain	Myalgia	Skin rash	Conjunctivitis	Periorbital edema	Chest pain	Arthralgia	Headache	Amyloidosis	CRP during attack (mg/dl)	CRP between attacks (mg/dl)	Other observations	Response to NSAID	Response to corticosteroid	Respond to etanercept	Respond to colchicine
8	8	T61I	G39V in *NLRP12*; Q49K in *PSMB8*	–	F	10	9–30	+	–	–	–	–	–	–	–	–	–	Slightly elevated	ND	Type1 diabetes mellitus, bilateral submandibular adenitis.	NA	NA	NA	NA
9	9	T61I	E721K in *PLCG2*; F402L in *NLRP12*; Q49K in *PSMB8*	–	F	5	14	+	–	+	–	–	–	–	–	–	–	11.5	7.0		ND	NA	NA	++
10	10	T61I	E84K/L110P/E148Q in *MEFV*	–	M	44	2	+	–	+	–	+	–	+	–	+	–				NA	NA	NA	NA
11	11	T61I	G39V in *NLRP12*; L70F in *NLRC4*	+	F	20	1	+	+	+	+	–	–	+	+	+	–	4.1	0.15		–	NA	–	–

Family	Case	*TNFRSF1A* variant	Variants in other genes	Family history	Gender	Age at onset, years	Duration of episode, days	Fever (>38 °C)	Abdominal pain	Myalgia	Skin rash	Conjunctivitis	Periorbital edema	Chest pain	Arthralgia	Headache	Amyloidosis	CRP during attack (mg/dl)	CRP between attacks (mg/dl)	Other observations	Response to NSAID	Response to corticosteroid	Respond to etanercept	Respond to colchicine
12	12	T61I	E148Q/E148Q/P369S/R408Q in *MEFV;* G39V in *NLRP12*; Q49K in *PSMB8*	–	M	28	90	+	–	+	+	+	–	–	+	–	–	5.5	0.04		–	NA	NA	++
13	13	T61I	E148Q/E148Q in *MEFV*	–	M	51	12	+	–	–	–	–	–	–	+	–	–	11.0	3.0	Cyclosporine was effective.	–	++	NA	+
14	14	T61I	M694I in *MEFV*	–	M	15	7–14	+	+	+	+	–	–	–	–	–	–	18.9	0.10	Splenomegaly, lymphadenopathy, hemophagocytic lymphohistiocytosis	+	–	NA	++
15	15	T61I	E148Q/M694I in *MEFV;* Q49K in *PSMB8*	+	F	17	14	+	+	–	–	–	–	+	–	+	–	15.1	0.07	Headache due to Tolosa-hunt syndrome	ND	+	NA	++

(continued)

Table 11.2 (continued)

Family	Case	*TNFRSF1A* variant	Variants in other genes	Family history	Gender	Age at onset, years	Duration of episode, days	Fever (>38 °C)	Abdominal pain	Myalgia	Skin rash	Conjunctivitis	Periorbital edema	Chest pain	Arthralgia	Headache	Amyloidosis	CRP during attack (mg/dl)	CRP between attacks (mg/dl)	Other observations	Response to NSAID	Response to corticosteroid	Respond to etanercept	Respond to colchicine
16	16	T61I	E148Q in *MEFV;* A612T in *NOD2;* Q49K in *PSMB8*	–	M	20	30–60	+	–	–	–	–	–	–	–	–	–	10.4	0.02	Hepatosplenomegaly	+	NA	NA	+
17	17	T61I	R471C in *NOD2*; Q49K in *PSMB8*	–	M	47	7	+	+	+	+	–	–	–	+	–	–	29.0	0.0	Shnitzler's syndrome	–	+	NA	++
18	18	T61I	G304R in *MEFV;* R471C in *NOD2*	–	F	32	0.5–5	+	–	+	–	–	–	+	+	+	–	1.4	0.06	SLE. Cyclosporine was effective.	+	+	NA	++
19	19	T61I	T335N in *PSTPIP1*	–	F	6	30–90	+	–	–	+	–	–	–	+	+	–	12.4	0.1	Neck tumor[b]	+	++	++	NA
20	20	C88Y	L110P/E148Q in *MEFV*	+	M	10	20	+	+	–	–	–	–	–	+	+	–	21.6	<0.04	Pharyngitis	+	++	NA	NA

Family	Case	*TNFRSF1A* variant	Variants in other genes	Family history	Gender	Age at onset, years	Duration of episode, days	Fever (>38 °C)	Abdominal pain	Myalgia	Skin rash	Conjunctivitis	Periorbital edema	Chest pain	Arthralgia	Headache	Amyloidosis	CRP during attack (mg/dl)	CRP between attacks (mg/dl)	Other observations	Response to NSAID	Response to corticosteroid	Respond to etanercept	Respond to colchicine
21	21	V125 M	ND	+	F	Childhood	Continuous	+	–	–	–	–	–	–	–	–	–	0.35	0.05	Cervical lymphadenopathy, parotid swelling, clavicle pain	–	+	[c]	NA
21	22	V125 M	ND	+	F	23	2–3	+	+	–	–	–	–	–	+	–	–	Negative	Negative		ND	+	+	NA
21	23	V125 M	ND	+	F	0.4	14	+	+	–	–	–	–	–	–	–	–	ND	ND		ND	ND	ND	ND
21	24	V125 M	ND	+	F	10	2–3	+	–	–	–	–	–	–	–	–	–	ND	ND		ND	ND	ND	ND
21	25	V125 M	ND	+	M	Childhood	7–10	+	–	–	–	–	–	–	–	–	–	ND	ND		ND	ND	ND	ND
22	26	V136 M	E148Q in *MEFV*	–	F	32	4–5	+	–	–	–	–	–	–	+	–	–	ND	Negative		+	NA	NA	NA
23	27	S321I	L110P/E148Q in *MEFV*	–	F	4	7–30	+	–	+	+	–	–		+	–	–	18.1	0.15		–	+	+	–

NA not administered, *ND* no data

Adapted from Clinical and genetic features of patients with TNFRSF1A variants in Japan: Findings of a nationwide survey. Arthritis Rheumatol. 2016;68:2760–2771

[a]Her sister had already been reported as TRAPS [35]. She was asymptomatic when her sister was reported

[b]Histopathology: inflammatory cell infiltration of the fibro-musculo-fatty-vascular tissue

[c]Discontinuation due to adverse event

Table 11.3 Genotype of patients with *TNFRSF1A* variants in Japan

TNFRSF1A variant	Family	Cases	Sporadic cases
C15Y[a]	1	1	1
N25D[a]	1	1	0
C30Y	2	3	0
C30R	1	3	0
T50M	2	3	0
T61I[a]	19	25	14
C70G	1	3	0
C70S[a]	1	3	0
C88Y	1	1	0
N101K[a]	1	1	1
V125M[a]	1	5	0
V136M[a]	1	1	1
S321I[a]	1	1	1
Total	33	51	18

Adapted from Clinical and genetic features of patients with TNFRSF1A variants in Japan: Findings of a nationwide survey. Arthritis Rheumatol. 2016;68:2760–2771.
[a]*TNFRSF1A* variants that had not been reported outside Japan.

parents of 1 patient each with the C15Y and S321I variants underwent genetic analysis. Both parents of 1 patient with the T61I variant was found to carry the variant, and 1 parent each of the other 6 patients carried the variant. De novo mutations were not found. The C15Y, N25D, T61I, C70S, N101K, V125M, V136M, and S321I variants were reported exclusively in Japan.

11.10 Clinical Features of Patients with TNFRSF1A Variant in Japan

The main clinical findings in Japanese patients with *TNFRSF1A* variants are a fever of 38 °C (100% of patients), abdominal pain (36%), myalgia (43%), skin rash (55%), conjunctivitis (18%), periorbital edema (9%), chest pain (14%), arthralgia (59%), and headache (23%). No patient had amyloidosis. None of the Japanese patients underwent any abdominal operation because of misdiagnosis. When we classified the C15Y, T50M, and C70S variants as “structural mutations,” N25D, T61I, N101K, V125M, V136M, and S321I variants as other mutations, there was no significant difference in clinical manifestations between patients carrying “structural mutations” and others, except for family history and age at onset. A positive family history of recurrent inflammatory episodes of unknown cause and a disease onset at age <20 years were significantly more frequent in patients carrying “structural mutations” than others (94.1% vs. 29.2% and 87.5% vs. 58.1%, each).

We compared clinical characteristics between patients in Japan and those registered in the Eurofever/EUROTRAPS international registry, the largest cohort of patients carrying *TNFRSF1A*, with patients from six European countries participating [24]. All of the patients in Japan showed a fever of 38 °C, which was significantly more prevalent than the case in Europe (100% vs. 84%). In contrast, a number of clinical symptoms were significantly less frequent in Japanese patients, including abdominal pain (36% vs. 70%), myalgia (43% vs. 70%), and amyloidosis (0% vs. 10%). Clinical symptoms may be milder in Japanese patients than in Caucasian patients. Interestingly, a national survey of FMF in Japan revealed that Japanese FMF patients had a lower prevalence of abdominal pain and amyloidosis than Mediterranean FMF patients [38]. The low prevalence of abdominal pain and amyloidosis in autoinflammatory diseases may be an ethnic characteristic of Japanese.

11.11 The Pathogenic Significance of the TNFRSF1A Variants in Japan

Although the most prominent genetic characteristic in Japanese patients with *TNFRSF1A* variants is the presence of the T61I variant, the most common variant in Japanese patients, the pathogenic significance of this variant remains unclear. In our 16 patients carrying the T61I variant, two patients had the M694I mutations of MEFV. Their inflammatory symptoms were explained with the M694I mutations of MEFV. We considered the possibility that patients carrying the T61I variant had other autoinflammatory disease-related gene mutations. We conducted genetic analysis of *NLRP3*, *NOD2*, *PSTPIP1*, *PLCG2*, *NLRP12*, *IL1RN*, *NLRC4*, and *PSMB8* in addition to *TNFRSF1A*, *MEFV*, and *MVK*. These additional eight genes are supposed to cover almost all of the genes responsible for autoinflammatory diseases [49–53]. In our 16 patients carrying the T61I variant (patients 4–19 in Table 11.2), we identified some additional variants. All variants except 1 were supposed to be common variants according to the Exome Aggregation Consortium database (http://exac.broadinstitute.org). Only patient 11 was carrying a rare *NLRC4* variant, L70F. Although *NLRC4* mutations that have been reported to cause autoinflammation are located in the nucleotide-binding oligomerization domain coding region, L70F is located in the caspase recruitment domain coding region [50–52]. Therefore, the pathogenic role of L70F is not clear. In our 16 patients carrying the T61I variant, except for two patients having the M694I mutations of *MEFV*, we identified no other pathogenic variants in a total of 11 autoinflammatory disease-related genes, which might support a possible pathogenic role of the T61I variant.

Two-thirds of the patients carrying the T61I variant had sporadic illness. There was no significant difference in the allele frequency of the T61I variant between patients and controls; however, there was a trend toward an increased frequency of the T61I variant in patients ($p = 0.071$). Considering that the sister of patient 6 was homozygous for the T61I variant but was asymptomatic (Table 11.2), it may be certain that the T61I variant does not have a potent pathogenic effect seen with "structural mutations." It is interesting that two patients having a combination of heterozygous T61I and heterozygous M694I mutations of MEFV had inflammatory episodes for up to 14 days, which is long compared to the typical FMF course, which terminates within 3 days. It is possible that the T61I variant influences the phenotype of the M694I mutation.

A small number of patients and none of healthy controls had the C15Y, N25D, N101K, V125M, V136M, and S321I variants. Therefore, their pathogenic significance could not be deduced from the penetrance level. We thought that it would be useful to examine the cell surface and intracellular expression of variant TNFRI proteins to assess their contribution to disease. We examined the effect on TNFRI trafficking of variants by using the same experimental procedures as those described previously [10]. We transfected expression vectors encoding wild-type or variant TNFRI into human embryonic 293T cells. We assessed the cell surface expression of receptors by using FACS analysis. Consistent with a previous observation, cells transfected with C33Y or T50M TNFRI showed less cell surface expression than cells transfected with wild-type or R92Q TNFRI. Cells transfected with the C15Y variant showed decreased cell surface expression, in the same manner as the C33Y and T50M variants. In contrast, cells transfected with N25D, T61I, N101K, V125M, V136M, and S321I receptors showed cell surface expression at levels as high as those in cells with the wild-type or R92Q receptor. This result suggests that the C15Y variant has the same pathogenic significance as the other "structural mutations." In contrast, the N25D, T61I, N101K, V125M, V136M, and S321I variants should be distinguished from "structural mutations."

11.12 Diagnostic Indicators of Japanese TRAPS

Because the rate of mutation detection is low (<20%) among patients having symptoms consistent with autoinflammatory diseases, A diagnostic score to predict the probability of a positive genetic test result for any of the *TNFRSF1A*, *MEFV*, and *MVK* genes has been proposed by Gattorno et al. [54]. Most of the patients in that study were children age < 18 years and of Italian origin, which is a different population from that of our patients. In addition, abdominal pain, which was less frequent in Japanese patients with *TNFRSF1A* variants, was included in the calculation as an important predicting factor. We therefore considered that this scoring system was not applicable to our patients.

In order to identify sensitive and specific markers for detecting *TNFRSF1A* mutations in our Japanese patients, the clinical features of the patients carrying *TNFRSF1A* "structural mutations" (n = 17) and those without any *TNFRSF1A* mutations/variants (n = 146) were compared to elucidate variables for obtaining positive results by genetic analysis of *TNFRSF1A*. Using univariate analyses, we identified a positive family history of recurrent inflammatory episodes of unknown cause and a disease onset at age <20 years as clinical parameters predicting positive results of genetic analysis. Multivariate logistic regression analysis showed that only a positive family history of recurrent inflammatory episodes was strongly associated with the possibility of obtaining a positive result for "structural mutation" of the *TNFRSF1A* gene. There were no significant differences in symptoms such as fever, abdominal pain, myalgia, and skin rash. In our Japanese cohort, when the patient had a family history of recurrent inflammatory episodes, the sensitivity was 94.1% and the specificity was 89.7% for the probability of carrying *TNFRSF1A* "structural mutations." Further validation of this finding is needed with another patient cohort.

On the basis of these results, TRAPS diagnostic criteria, which are conditions for certification of designated intractable diseases "Nanbyo" and chronic specific diseases for children, were created. By satisfying this, patients can receive public medical expense subsidies. Repeated symptoms of inflammation more than 6 months are essential conditions and genetic testing is recommended when satisfying supplementary items such as family history. The final diagnosis is by genetic testing. Interpretation of genetic test results requires consultation with experts.

11.13 Conclusion

We conducted a nationwide survey for TRAPS for the first time in Japan or Asia overall. The incidence of patients with *TNFRSF1A* variants in Japan was rare, as in other European countries, but a number of clinical and genetic features of Japanese patients were different from those of Caucasian patients.

Many of the *TNFRSF1A* variants identified in Japan, including the T61I variant, have an uncertain pathogenic significance. It is considered essential for the understanding of Japanese TRAPS to clarify the pathogenic significance of these variants.

References

1. Hull KM, Drewe E, Aksentijevich I, Singh HK, Wong K, Mcdermott EM, et al. The TNF receptor-associated periodic syndrome (TRAPS). Medicine. 2002;81:349–68. https://doi.org/10.1097/00005792-200209000-00002.
2. Ueda N, Ida H, Washio M, Miyahara H, Tokunaga S, Tanaka F, et al. Clinical and genetic features of patients with TNFRSF1A variants in Japan: findings of a Nationwide survey. Arthritis & Rheumatology. 2016;68:2760–71. https://doi.org/10.1002/art.39793.
3. Masters SL, Simon A, Aksentijevich I, Kastner DL. Horror Autoinflammaticus: the molecular pathophysiology of autoinflammatory disease. Annu Rev Immunol. 2009;27:621–68. https://doi.org/10.1146/annurev.immunol.25.022106.141627.
4. Mulley J, Saar K, Hewitt G, Rüschendorf F, Phillips H, Colley A, et al. Gene localization for an autosomal dominant familial periodic fever to 12p13. Am J Hum Genet. 1998;62:884–9. https://doi.org/10.1086/301793.
5. Mcdermott MF, Ogunkolade BW, Mcdermott EM, Jones LC, Wan Y, Quane KA, et al. Linkage of familial Hibernian fever to chromosome 12p13. Am J Hum Genet. 1998;62:1446–51. https://doi.org/10.1086/301886.

6. Mcdermott MF, Aksentijevich I, Galon J, Mcdermott EM, Ogunkolade B, Centola M, et al. Germline mutations in the extracellular domains of the 55 kDa TNF receptor, TNFR1, define a family of dominantly inherited autoinflammatory syndromes. Cell. 1999;97:133–44. https://doi.org/10.1016/s0092-8674(00)80721-7.
7. Banner DW, D'Arcy A, Janes W, Gentz R, Schoenfeld HJ, Broger C, et al. Crystal structure of the soluble human 55 kd TNF receptor-human TNF beta complex: implications for TNF receptor activation. Cell. 1993;73:431–45. https://doi.org/10.2210/pdb1tnr/pdb.
8. Chan FK, Chun HJ, Zheng L, Siegel RM, Bui KL, Lenardo MJ. A domain in TNF receptors that mediates ligand-independent receptor assembly and signaling. Science. 2000;288:2351–4. https://doi.org/10.1126/science.288.5475.2351.
9. Hawari FI, Rouhani FN, Cui X, Yu Z-X, Buckley C, Kaler M, et al. Release of full-length 55-kDa TNF receptor 1 in exosome-like vesicles: a mechanism for generation of soluble cytokine receptors. Proc Natl Acad Sci. 2004;101:1297–302. https://doi.org/10.1073/pnas.0307981100.
10. Lobito AA, Kimberley FC, Muppidi JR, Komarow H, Jackson AJ, Hull KM, et al. Abnormal disulfide-linked oligomerization results in ER retention and altered signaling by TNFR1 mutants in TNFR1-associated periodic fever syndrome (TRAPS). Blood. 2006;108:1320–7. https://doi.org/10.1182/blood-2005-11-006783.
11. Simon A, Park H, Maddipati R, Lobito AA, Bulua AC, Jackson AJ, et al. Concerted action of wild-type and mutant TNF receptors enhances inflammation in TNF receptor 1-associated periodic fever syndrome. Proc Natl Acad Sci. 2010;107:9801–6. https://doi.org/10.1073/pnas.0914118107.
12. Bachetti T, Chiesa S, Castagnola P, Bani D, Zanni ED, Omenetti A, et al. Autophagy contributes to inflammation in patients with TNFR-associated periodic syndrome (TRAPS). Ann Rheum Dis. 2012;72:1044–52. https://doi.org/10.1136/annrheumdis-2012-201952.
13. Bulua AC, Simon A, Maddipati R, Pelletier M, Park H, Kim KY, et al. Mitochondrial reactive oxygen species promote production of proinflammatory cytokines and are elevated in TNFR1-associated periodic syndrome (TRAPS). J Exp Med. 2011;208:519–33. https://doi.org/10.1084/jem.20102049.
14. Dickie LJ, Aziz AM, Savic S, Lucherini OM, Cantarini L, Geiler J, et al. Involvement of X-box binding protein 1 and reactive oxygen species pathways in the pathogenesis of tumour necrosis factor receptor-associated periodic syndrome. Ann Rheum Dis. 2012;71:2035–43. https://doi.org/10.1136/annrheumdis-2011-201197.
15. Ravet N, Rouaghe S, Dode C, Bienvenu J, Stirnemann J, Levy P, et al. Clinical significance of P46L and R92Q substitutions in the tumour necrosis factor superfamily 1A gene. Ann Rheum Dis. 2006;65:1158–62. https://doi.org/10.1136/ard.2005.048611.
16. Tchernitchko D, Chiminqgi M, Galactéros F, Préhu C, Segbena Y, Coulibaly H, et al. Unexpected high frequency of P46L TNFRSF1A allele in sub-Saharan west African populations. Eur J Hum Genet. 2004;13:513–5. https://doi.org/10.1038/sj.ejhg.5201344.
17. Dosualdo A, Ferlito F, Prigione I, Obici L, Meini A, Zulian F, et al. Neutrophils from patients withTNFRSF1A mutations display resistance to tumor necrosis factor–induced apoptosis: Pathogenetic and clinical implications. Arthritis Rheum. 2006;54:998–1008. https://doi.org/10.1002/art.21657.
18. Aksentijevich I, Galon J, Soares M, Mansfield E, Hull K, Oh HH, et al. The tumor-necrosis-factor receptor-associated periodic syndrome: new mutations in TNFRSF1A, ancestral origins, genotype-phenotype studies, and evidence for further genetic heterogeneity of periodic fevers. Am J Hum Genet. 2001;69:301–14. https://doi.org/10.1086/321976.
19. Dieude P, Goossens M, Cornelis F, Michou L, Bardin T, Tchernitchko DO. The TNFRSF1A R92Q mutation is frequent in rheumatoid arthritis but shows no evidence for association or linkage with the disease. Ann Rheum Dis. 2007;66:1113–5. https://doi.org/10.1136/ard.2006.060764.

20. Amoura Z, Dodé C, Hue S, Caillat-Zucman S, Bahram S, Delpech M, et al. Association of the R92QTNFRSF1Amutation and extracranial deep vein thrombosis in patients with Behçets disease. Arthritis Rheum. 2005;52:608–11. https://doi.org/10.1002/art.20873.
21. Poirier O, Nicaud V, Gariépy J, Courbon D, Elbaz A, Morrison C, et al. Polymorphism R92Q of the tumour necrosis factor receptor 1 gene is associated with myocardial infarction and carotid intima-media thickness – the ECTIM, AXA, EVA and GENIC studies. Eur J Hum Genet. 2003;12:213–9. https://doi.org/10.1038/sj.ejhg.5201143.
22. Cantarini L, Lucherini OM, Brucato A, Barone L, Cumetti D, Iacoponi F, et al. Clues to detect tumor necrosis factor receptor-associated periodic syndrome (TRAPS) among patients with idiopathic recurrent acute pericarditis: results of a multicentre study. Clin Res Cardiol. 2012;101:525–31. https://doi.org/10.1007/s00392-012-0422-8.
23. Jager PLD, Jia X, Wang J, Bakker PIWD, Ottoboni L, Aggarwal NT, et al. Meta-analysis of genome scans and replication identify CD6, IRF8 and TNFRSF1A as new multiple sclerosis susceptibility loci. Nat Genet. 2009;41:776–82. https://doi.org/10.1038/ng.401.
24. Lachmann HJ, Papa R, Gerhold K, Obici L, Touitou I, Cantarini L, et al. The phenotype of TNF receptor-associated autoinflammatory syndrome (TRAPS) at presentation: a series of 158 cases from the Eurofever/EUROTRAPS international registry. Ann Rheum Dis. 2013;73:2160–7. https://doi.org/10.1136/annrheumdis-2013-204184.
25. Kallinich T. "periodic fever" without fever: two cases of non-febrile TRAPS with mutations in the TNFRSF1A gene presenting with episodes of inflammation or monosymptomatic amyloidosis. Ann Rheum Dis. 2005;65:958–60. https://doi.org/10.1136/ard.2005.043570.
26. Aganna E, Hammond L, Hawkins PN, Aldea A, McKee SA, van Amstel HK, et al. Heterogeneity among patients with tumor necrosis factor receptor-associated periodic syndrome phenotypes. Arthritis Rheum. 2003;48:2632–44. https://doi.org/10.1002/art.11215.
27. Kusuhara K, Hoshina T, Saito M, Ishimura M, Inoue H, Horiuchi T, et al. Successful treatment of a patient with tumor necrosis factor receptor-associated periodic syndrome using a half-dose of etanercept. Pediatr Int. 2012;54:552–5. https://doi.org/10.1111/j.1442-200x.2011.03525.x.
28. ter Haar NM, Oswald M, Jeyaratnam J, Anton J, Barron KS, Brogan PA, et al. Recommendations for the management of autoinflammatory diseases. Ann Rheum Dis. 2015;74:1636–44. https://doi.org/10.1136/annrheumdis-2015-207546.
29. Gattorno M, Obici L, Cattalini M, Tormey V, Abrams K, Davis N, et al. Canakinumab treatment for patients with active recurrent or chronic TNF receptor-associated periodic syndrome (TRAPS): an open-label, phase II study. Ann Rheum Dis. 2016;76:173–8. https://doi.org/10.1136/annrheumdis-2015-209031.
30. Bulua AC, Mogul DB, Aksentijevich I, Singh H, He DY, Muenz LR, et al. Efficacy of etanercept in the tumor necrosis factor receptor-associated periodic syndrome: a prospective, open-label, dose-escalation study. Arthritis Rheum. 2012;64:908–13. https://doi.org/10.1002/art.33416.
31. Jacobelli S, Andre M, Alexandra J-F, Dode C, Papo T. Failure of anti-TNF therapy in TNF receptor 1-associated periodic syndrome (TRAPS). Rheumatology. 2007;46:1211–2. https://doi.org/10.1093/rheumatology/kel298.
32. Drewe E, Powell R, Mcdermott E. Comment on: failure of anti-TNF therapy in TNF receptor 1-associated periodic syndrome (TRAPS). Rheumatology. 2007;46:1865–6. https://doi.org/10.1093/rheumatology/kem231.
33. Siebert S, Amos N, Lawson TM. Comment on: failure of anti-TNF therapy in TNF receptor 1-associated periodic syndrome (TRAPS). Rheumatology. 2007;47:228–9. https://doi.org/10.1093/rheumatology/kem243.
34. Lainka E, Neudorf U, Lohse P, Timmann C, Stojanov S, Huss K, et al. Incidence of TNFRSF1A mutations in German children: epidemiological, clinical and genetic characteristics. Rheumatology. 2009;48:987–91. https://doi.org/10.1093/rheumatology/kep140.
35. Kusuhara K, Nomura A, Nakao F, Hara T. Tumour necrosis factor receptor-associated periodic syndrome with a novel mutation in the TNFRSF1A gene in a Japanese family. Eur J Pediatr. 2004;163:30–2. https://doi.org/10.1007/s00431-003-1338-0.

36. Washio M, Nakano T, Kawaguchi Y, Takagi K, Kiyohara C, Tsukamoto H, et al. Tumor necrosis factor receptor-associated periodic syndrome (TRAPS) in Japan: a review of the literature. Mod Rheumatol. 2013;23:210–7. https://doi.org/10.3109/s10165-012-0737-3.
37. Tsuchiya-Suzuki A, Yazaki M, Nakamura A, Yamazaki K, Agematsu K, Matsuda M, et al. Clinical and genetic features of familial Mediterranean fever in Japan. J Rheumatol. 2009;36:1671–6. https://doi.org/10.3899/jrheum.081278.
38. Migita K, Uehara R, Nakamura Y, Yasunami M, Tsuchiya-Suzuki A, Yazaki M, et al. Familial Mediterranean fever in Japan. Medicine (Baltimore). 2012;91:337–43. https://doi.org/10.1097/MD.0b013e318277cf75.
39. Manki A, Nishikomori R, Nakata-Hizume M, Kunitomi T, Takei S, Urakami T, et al. Tumor necrosis factor receptor-associated periodic syndrome mimicking systemic juvenile idiopathic arthritis. Allergol Int. 2006;55:337–41. https://doi.org/10.2332/allergolint.55.337.
40. Livneh A, Langevitz P, Zemer D, Zaks N, Kees S, Lidar T, et al. Criteria for the diagnosis of familial mediterranean fever. Arthritis Rheum. 1997;40:1879–85. https://doi.org/10.1002/art.1780401023.
41. Ida H. A novel mutation (T61I) in the gene encoding tumour necrosis factor receptor superfamily 1A (TNFRSF1A) in a Japanese patient with tumour necrosis factor receptor-associated periodic syndrome (TRAPS) associated with systemic lupus erythematosus. Rheumatology. 2004;43:1292–9. https://doi.org/10.1093/rheumatology/keh320.
42. Horiuchi T, Tsukamoto H, Mitoma H, Miyagawa H, Tamimoto Y, Yoshizawa S, et al. Novel mutations in TNFRSF1A in patients with typical tumor necrosis factor receptor-associated periodic syndrome and with systemic lupus erythematosus in Japanese. Int J Mol Med. 2004. https://doi.org/10.3892/ijmm.14.5.813.
43. Ohmori S, Hino R, Nakamura M, Tokura Y. Heparin serves as a natural stimulant of the inflammasome and exacerbates the symptoms of tumor necrosis factor receptor-associated periodic syndrome (TRAPS). J Dermatol Sci. 2012;66:82–4. https://doi.org/10.1016/j.jdermsci.2011.11.006.
44. Ohmori S, Hino R, Nakamura M. Inflammatory response to heparinoid and heparin in a patient with tumor necrosis factor receptor-associated periodic syndrome: the second case with a T61I mutation in theTNFRSF1Agene. J Dermatol. 2014;41:1112–3. https://doi.org/10.1111/1346-8138.12689.
45. Takagi K, Kawaguchi Y, Fujikawa S, Otani T, Sugiura T, Hara M. Tumor necrosis factor receptor-associated periodic syndrome with a C30R mutation in a Japanese family. Mod Rheumatol. 2007;17:265–6. https://doi.org/10.1007/s10165-007-0580-0.
46. Kai M, Tamaki S, Nishikomori R, Takaoka Y, Ohara O, Oshima K. A case of TNF receptor-associated periodic syndrome. Ryumachika (Rheumatology). 2011;45:456–460. In Japanese.
47. Nakamura M. Tokura Y. A novel missense mutation in tumour necrosis factor receptor superfamily 1A (TNFRSF1A) gene found in tumour necrosis factor receptor-associated periodic syndrome (TRAPS) with high serum interleukin (IL)-22. Eur J Dermatol. 2010;20:508–9. https://doi.org/10.1684/ejd.2010.0951.
48. Nakamura M, Kobayashi M, Tokura Y. A novel missense mutation in tumour necrosis factor receptor superfamily 1A (TNFRSF1A) gene found in tumour necrosis factor receptor-associated periodic syndrome (TRAPS) manifesting adult-onset still disease-like skin eruptions: report of a case and review of the Japanese patients. Br J Dermatol. 2009;161:968–70. https://doi.org/10.1111/j.1365-2133.2009.09409.x.
49. Zhou Q, Lee GS, Brady J, Datta S, Katan M, Sheikh A, et al. A hypermorphic missense mutation in PLCG2, encoding phospholipase Cγ2, causes a dominantly inherited autoinflammatory disease with immunodeficiency. Am J Hum Genet. 2012;91:713–20. https://doi.org/10.1016/j.ajhg.2012.08.006.
50. Romberg N, Moussawi KA, Nelson-Williams C, Stiegler AL, Loring E, Choi M, et al. Mutation of NLRC4 causes a syndrome of enterocolitis and autoinflammation. Nat Genet. 2014;46:1135–9. https://doi.org/10.1038/ng.3066.

51. Canna SW, Jesus AAD, Gouni S, Brooks SR, Marrero B, Liu Y, et al. An activating NLRC4 inflammasome mutation causes autoinflammation with recurrent macrophage activation syndrome. Nat Genet. 2014;46:1140–6. https://doi.org/10.1038/ng.3089.
52. Kitamura A, Sasaki Y, Abe T, Kano H, Yasutomo K. An inherited mutation inNLRC4causes autoinflammation in human and mice. J Exp Med. 2014;211:2385–96. https://doi.org/10.1084/jem.20141091.
53. Arima K, Kinoshita A, Mishima H, Kanazawa N, Kaneko T, Mizushima T, et al. Proteasome assembly defect due to a proteasome subunit beta type 8 (PSMB8) mutation causes the autoinflammatory disorder, Nakajo-Nishimura syndrome. Proc Natl Acad Sci. 2011;108:14914–9. https://doi.org/10.1073/pnas.1106015108.
54. Gattorno M, Sormani MP, Dosualdo A, Pelagatti MA, Caroli F, Federici S, et al. A diagnostic score for molecular analysis of hereditary autoinflammatory syndromes with periodic fever in children. Arthritis Rheum. 2008;58:1823–32. https://doi.org/10.1002/art.23474.

MIX
Papier aus verantwortungsvollen Quellen
Paper from responsible sources
FSC® C105338

If you have any concerns about our products,
you can contact us on
ProductSafety@springernature.com

In case Publisher is established outside the EU,
the EU authorized representative is:
Springer Nature Customer Service Center GmbH
Europaplatz 3, 69115 Heidelberg, Germany

Printed by Libri Plureos GmbH
in Hamburg, Germany